# Mental Illness and the Bo

Observation of the body helps psychiatrists to determine the cause and treatment of mental illness. To form a diagnosis, practitioners conduct detailed observations of a patient's appearance, posture, gesture and gait, thereby using the body as a diagnostic index. However, within routine mental health practice, there is little consideration of how the bodily presentation of patients may reflect aspects of their 'lived experience'.

With reference to a range of theoretical perspectives including philosophy, psychoanalysis, feminism and sociology, *Mental Illness and the Body* explores the ways in which understanding 'lived experience' may usefully be applied to mental health practice. Key features include:

- an overview of the history of British psychiatry including treatments
- an analysis of feminism and the way its insights have been applied to understanding women's mental health and illness
- in-depth interviews with four patients diagnosed with mental illness
- an outline of Freudian and post-Freudian perspectives on the body and their relevance to current mental health practice.

*Mental Illness and the Body* is essential reading for mental health practitioners, allied professionals and anyone with an interest in the body and mental illness.

**Louise Phillips** is a lecturer in Mental Health at City University and a mental health nurse. She has practiced for the past 19 years in a variety of settings including elderly care, the voluntary sector and the NHS. Prior to starting her academic career, she worked for a number of years as a Community Psychiatric Nurse in the King's Cross area of London. In addition to her nursing qualification she has a BA in European Cultural History and completed her PhD on approaches to the body and mental illness at the University of Kent at Canterbury in 2003.

# Mental Illness and the Body

## Beyond diagnosis

## Louise Phillips

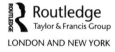

Routledge
Taylor & Francis Group

LONDON AND NEW YORK

First published 2006
by Routledge
2 Park Square, Milton Park, Abingdon, Oxon OX14 4RN

Simultaneously published in the USA and Canada
by Routledge
270 Madison Avenue, New York, NY 10016

*Routledge is an imprint of the Taylor & Francis Group, an informa business*

© 2006 Louise Phillips

Typeset in Times New Roman by
Florence Production Ltd, Stoodleigh, Devon
Printed and bound in Great Britain by
The Cromwell Press, Trowbridge, Wiltshire

*British Library Cataloguing in Publication Data*
A catalogue record for this book is available
from the British Library

*Library of Congress Cataloging in Publication Data*
A catalog record for this book has been requested

ISBN10: 0-415-38320-x (hbk)
ISBN10: 0-415-38321-8 (pbk)
ISBN10: 0-203-08863-8 (ebk)

ISBN13: 978-0-415-38320-2 (hbk)
ISBN13: 978-0-415-38321-9 (pbk)
ISBN13: 978-0-203-08863-0 (ebk)

*Energy is the only life and is from the body.*
William Blake, *The Marriage of Heaven and Hell*

# Contents

# Acknowledgements

I would like to acknowledge the eight patients (four of whom are presented in this book) at the day hospital for generously allowing me to interview and observe them, and forming the basis of my research. Also, to the staff team for making me welcome. I am very grateful to my PhD supervisor Professor Janet Sayers for her guidance. Also to Geoff Brennan and Karen Bowler for reading the first draft. Thanks to friends and colleagues at City University for time and encouragement to complete first, my PhD, and then this book. Thanks also to Rachel Richardson who very kindly accompanied me several times around the grounds where Long Grove Hospital once was, and evoking many memories of the patients I first worked with. Many thanks to Marie-Laure Davenport. I would also like to mention my partner Rob, for making me laugh during the production of the manuscript, and whose love and encouragement helped make it possible.

# Preface

I trained as a mental health nurse in a 'mental asylum' called Long Grove Hospital (opened in 1907) in Epsom, Surrey. I lived in the nursing home located in the hospital grounds for four years, first as a student nurse and then, for a year, as a staff nurse on Ward 'A' (a chronic long stay ward for men, where they seemed to allocate all 'rebellious' newly qualified nurses). Prior to the introduction of the university-based Project 2000 course, Registered Mental Nurse training as it was then called, often took place in old hospitals that were situated on the outskirts of towns. There were five large hospitals surrounding Epsom and the grounds were vast and beautiful. At Long Grove, there was an adjoining farm (where prior to the 1970s, patients performed 'therapeutic' work) and a cherry orchard. Several unusual shrubs were transferred into the grounds of the hospital, for their protection from bomb damage, from Kew Botanical Gardens during the Second World War. My great grandfather was actually head gardener at Long Grove and my grandmother used to tell me how she visited him there and described encountering some 'odd' people along the way.

Among my most colourful and moving memories of that time are those of the many people who were patients there. One of the advantages of the 'old style' nurse training was that, as students, our first placement took place on an acute ward, which meant we were thrown in at the deep end. Then, following this, the training was organised so that we were given an opportunity to encounter a variety of clinical areas: rehabilitation, elderly care, community and a 'special' placement consisting of work with either alcoholics (which was my placement), adolescents, drug addicts or private patients experiencing neurotic conditions.

I remember many of the patients I worked with during my training and recall feeling intrigued by their descriptions of their lives. One woman felt that fashion designers, whose work was displayed in the 'fashion boutiques' in Oxford Street, had stolen her design ideas. She told me how before entering hospital she would walk along Oxford Street angrily looking at the clothes carefully arranged on mannequins. A male patient had become paranoid about his brother getting hold of his father's wealth. He thought his brother had devised a clever plan, which nobody else would be able to make sense of, in order to acquire the money. This idea preoccupied him so intently that he used a bow and arrow to shoot his brother who was gardening at the time. A sixty-two year old woman patient consistently played the Beatles song 'Dizzy Miss Lizzy' very loudly, and proudly stated she was just sixteen. Another woman kept repeating that she was in bed with her boyfriend when 'the fucking roof blew off'.

I'm in danger here, I know, of celebrating the so-called 'creative madness' of these people. However, most of all, I was intrigued by the way my first patients looked. I was interested in the ways in which they held themselves, how they walked, and their gestures. Some people were grimacing, reaching at invisible things in the air, scratching themselves and making their skin sore. Other people were flicking things away with their fingers, smacking themselves or holding their limbs in apparently uncomfortable positions.

My teachers at Long Grove informed me that the gestures of patients were the result of 'mental illness' and in particular 'schizophrenia', which was caused by too much of a particular chemical called dopamine in the brain. This appeared to be the only explanation. 'They' can see things that aren't there, I was told. They can hear voices when nobody is saying anything and they think that 'alien' things are inside them, or coming after them. Of course, on reflection nearly twenty years later, many of the gestures I observed in many patients, may indeed have been the result of brain chemical imbalance. They were also indicative of side effects of some of the older forms of anti-psychotic medication. 'Extrapyramidal' symptoms produced tongue protrusion, lip smacking, chewing, blinking, foot tapping and shoulder shrugging. 'Akinesia' induced side effects such as a mask-like face, a shuffling walk, muscle stiffness and so on. The gestures of people with mental illness were merely reduced to biological explanations. Yet, I was interested in something that was not directly related to medication or brain chemicals. I felt that people were perhaps expressing, willingly or unwillingly, something about their lives, and that this was not being considered.

Years later, I decided I would explore this further. The acknowledgement and respect of patients' bodily gestures, and the possible meaning inherent in them, became the focus of a PhD thesis, which I completed in 2003. This thesis then became the foundation of this book. The PhD thesis consisted of eight case studies of people diagnosed with mental illness and, for the purposes of this book, I have selected four (outlined in Chapter 8). In the case studies, I provide a brief biographical background to each person. I describe my observations of, and interactions with, these people in terms of their bodily presentation, including my responses. I then offer my interpretation of the meanings apparent in their bodies in terms of their life experiences.

In the day hospital where I conducted this research, I left some information/leaflets about the study for patients to respond to. I felt it was more appropriate for patients to choose to come forward if they felt comfortable about being observed and about speaking to me about their experiences of their bodies, rather than me randomly selecting them to do so. My research was not representative of a large group or population. It was based on those patients attending the day hospital who chose to come forward. As part of my role as lecturer in mental health nursing, I attended the day hospital weekly as my clinical contact area. I felt that through my continuing contact with patients, I was well placed to conduct my research. I have changed the names of the people presented in the case studies in this book.

Long Grove was closed in 1992 following the introduction – perceived by some as unwelcome – of Care in the Community. Long-term patients were moved into 'ordinary' hostels and houses in an effort to 'normalise' them and integrate them into the community. The patients at Long Grove were moved to inner-city areas with low property values. In his book about the closure of Long Grove, Tony Day movingly describes how a Polish Second World War survivor refused to leave his home: 'the ward, now empty of furniture, was locked. Everybody else was gone, but he continued to wander Long Grove's empty corridors' (1993: 112). This person did eventually leave of course, but along with the other patients of Long Grove, he was no longer able to enjoy its beautiful grounds. Long Grove now consists of a collection of about 300 luxury houses and flats. In fact, some of the old buildings of the hospital are still there. Many of the wards, including the main hospital building (where the doctors stayed), have been converted into flats. I recently visited this site and experienced vivid memories of my experiences there. This book is dedicated to those patients who, upon reflection, first inspired me to write this book.

# Chapter 1

# Introduction

Some years after leaving Long Grove, I worked in a registered care home for people diagnosed with severe mental illness who had been moved out of other large asylums. I worked closely with one particular patient I will call Marilyn. She was fifty-two and a long-standing patient who had been regularly hospitalised since her twenties. Like the other residents, Marilyn came to live in this particular home because the large institution where she formally lived was closing. Marilyn did not want to leave the institution and was sedated and driven in an ambulance to the registered care home. On arrival she was very distressed. She was verbally aggressive towards staff and other residents, and among numerous examples of disturbed behaviour, Marilyn would regularly lift her clothes to pee on the carpet next to a window in full view of people outside waiting at a bus stop.

Due to the severity of her psychiatric symptoms, Marilyn was prescribed a relatively new anti-psychotic medication called Clozaril and her behaviour became more settled. However, following this intervention, which was considered highly successful by clinicians, other forms of behaviour came to the fore. She consistently refused to wear day clothes or to leave the confines of her home stating that if she did she would be sucked into the sky. Similarly, Marilyn refused to bathe for fear of being sucked down the plughole, resulting in her becoming very unkempt and developing a strong body odour. As she washed infrequently and perspired so much, she developed a painful rash under her breasts and around her groin. She pulled out her hair from the top of her head, leaving a fine downy scalp that was complemented by long and greasy side locks. She carried several bags with her around the house, which appeared to be stuffed full of tissues, clothes and bits of paper. She was very protective of these bags and did not let them out of her sight. Every day, Marilyn sat at the same chair in the dining room in a state of restlessness, smoking nervously and asking staff and other residents how they were getting on. Frequently, following visits by her mother, she giggled to herself, responding to such outbursts by exclaiming 'naughty girl' and smacking herself on the arm. Also she picked her nose, lining up her bogies in little balls on the dining room table.

In staff team meetings much emphasis was placed upon Marilyn. Understandably, the staff were concerned about her personal hygiene, physical appearance and domestic cleanliness. The clinicians responsible for her care focused upon Marilyn's body in terms of citing an imbalance of chemicals in her brain as a causative factor to her mental distress and consequent behaviour. Yet, I was struck by how little emphasis was placed upon Marilyn's body by both staff and visiting mental health professionals in terms of the possible meanings and significance attached to its very stark expression. No emphasis was placed upon what Marilyn's body indicated in terms of her *lived* experience. I wondered what Marilyn's bodily presentation was about and whether it extended beyond a mere manifestation of her mental illness. I wondered if Marilyn's body and its surroundings might express in some way aspects of her internal world. Might it be that she was unable to verbalise emotional distress and therefore used her body as a way of expressing it? Or might her body express something about her being a woman in the world? Did her body in some way represent an articulated resistance against societal conventions of femininity? What did her body say about her life? It was possible to look *beyond diagnosis.*

Bodies are fascinating. They are functional and biological entities, yet at the same time bodies depict aspects of the emotional self. It seems as if a person's experiences are contained within the physicality of their bodies. I remember as a child being fascinated by the famous escapologist Harry Houdini (1874–1926). I read how he would be contained within chains or submerged under water in locked crates. He would constrict his muscles and then use them to wriggle his way out of the impossible-to-escape spaces. He once said that his mind was the most effective key, but rumour has it that he often had a real one. As a teenager, I recall watching the uncoordinated and disconnected limbs of Ian Curtis of Joy Division, frenetically dancing while performing 'She's Lost Control'.

The depictions of bodies in art are especially enchanting when they seem to reflect the person being represented as inside out. My personal favourites include the paintings of Francis Bacon (1909–1992). In *Triptych* (1972) Bacon depicts his partner, George Dyer, who had died suddenly a year before, on the left section. The heart of this figure is not just broken; it has sunken and dropped out of the body and lays splattered on the floor. A big space is left where the heart once was. The nude bodies depicted within the paintings of Lucian Freud who was born in 1922 (I will deal with the work of his grandfather, Sigmund, largely in this book) reveal in the very texture of people's skin, as he has said, how people happen to be. His paintings are largely autobiographical, consisting of friends, family, lovers and so on.

The body is, of course, something that is essentially biological and functional. This 'material' perception of the body can be located within the disciplines of the natural sciences, law and medicine. Consisting of bones, nerves, ligaments, flesh and blood, our bodies enable most of us to function in the world. Our bodies are also vulnerable to the effects of ageing (and, of course, we are constantly encouraged to delay this process), illness and eventual death. There is another consideration of the body, which can be understood as 'discursive'. In this context, as Jane Ussher asserts, the body also exists as a site of discourse, as the representation of desire and fantasy and of signs and signifiers (1997: 1). Discursive approaches to the body are situated within the academic disciplines of sociology, psychoanalysis, philosophy and feminism.

## The body and mental health practice

The body is fundamentally relevant to mental health practice. British psychiatry has historically approached the cause and treatment of mental illness through observation of the body. This tradition continues within current psychiatric and allied mental health practice in the case of mental health assessment. To form a diagnosis, practitioners routinely conduct detailed observations of patients' appearance, posture, gesture and gait, thereby using the body as a diagnostic index. However, within the biomedical framework of routine mental health practice, there is little scope for considering how the bodily presentation of patients may reflect aspects of their lived experience. This book will suggest that it is useful to consider the meaning behind the gestures, expressions and gait of people experiencing mental illness. These expressions, perhaps, tell us that a person's experiences are very much present and relevant.

Within professional discourse and practice, there are a number of terms that are used to describe the phenomenon of mental illness. Throughout the book, I will be using the term 'mental illness', which, for me personally, is not an accurate term to describe the people I have worked with. It is rather difficult, however, to think of a term that best describes how some people appear to be attempting to relate their experiences and perceptions to others in a way that the rest of us might find bizarre, frightening and strange. The term 'mental *disorder*' is also open to controversy. It implies that there exists a mental *order* indicating a state of normality. In contrast, a disorder suggests abnormality. 'Mental distress' is perhaps not adequate either, as people are often not distressed as a result of their 'delusional' (for example) experiences.

As I often tell my students, as a teacher of 'mental health' and having worked in the field for nineteen years, I am still unclear as to what mental illness actually is. In terms of psychosis – which is the 'mental illness' I will be dealing with mostly in this book – there are certain experiences I have identified in the people I have worked with. People with psychosis (and I prefer to use this term rather than schizophrenia) seem to have some difficulty distinguishing between inside and outside, and seem to feel that parts of them are located within things outside of them. There seems to be a feeling of fragmentation and of being invaded from the outside or of invading objects in the outside world. There is often flatness in mood. I feel that the person experiencing what we call psychosis is perhaps willingly or unwillingly attempting to communicate their experiences in the world. Mainstream mental health practice, however, tends to regard these symptoms as meaningless and solely the result of organic mental illness. There are also a number of terms used to describe a person experiencing mental illness such as 'client', 'patient', 'service user' and so on. In this book, I will be using the term 'patient' to describe a person diagnosed with a mental illness.

I have observed in the many patients I have worked with who have a diagnosis of psychosis, that the use of words to express distress is often difficult, or even ineffective. This raises the question of how distress is articulated by language. Perhaps we all express distress through our actions and behaviour. We often use metaphors and clichés to express distress. We moan, cry or wail because we perhaps feel there are no words to communicate intense emotional pain. Perhaps we can say that certain ways of 'behaving' are possible indicators or metaphors for distress. Some actions are considered as 'normal' and acceptable, while others are deemed as bizarre and strange, as in the case of psychosis. If language is not an effective way of communicating distress, the body itself seems to take on the role of communicator of what that person has experienced or is experiencing.

## What this book does not do

In the four case studies I present in Chapter 8, the people all have a diagnosis of psychosis. In addition, they also experience anxiety and depression, and in the case of Alice, alcohol abuse. This book does not cover eating disorders or self-harm. There is already a wealth of information of psychological understandings of these conditions.[1] However, the two women I discuss in the case studies have both experienced difficulties with eating. There are also other psychiatric conditions relating closely to the body. These include Body Dysmorphic Disorder[2] and psychosomatic disorders. I mention these two conditions in my review of psychiatric texts in Chapter 3, but there has been discussion about the psychological explanations for these forms of distress that I do not cover in this book. Joyce McDougall in *Theatres of the Body: A Psychoanalytic Approach to Psychosomatic Illness* (1989) for example, provides several case studies of people who present with psychosomatic illness in the form of physical symptoms such as pain, anxiety and insomnia that have no apparent medical cause.

McDougall states that these 'symptoms' are a person's way of coping with life. She demonstrates that symptoms often disappear when the person is able to verbalise their distress. McDougall is, herself, a psychoanalyst and directs her understandings – and her valuable recommendations in terms of clinical practice – to the psychoanalysis profession. However, there have been no books specifically written for mental health practitioners that directly address the body and its presentation[3] in the understanding and treatment of mental illness.

## Overview of this book

The concept of 'lived experience' is firmly located in a philosophical tradition, which I briefly discuss in Chapter 2. I outline the tradition of phenomenology including the work of Merleau-Ponty and his development of the concept of the 'lived body'. I state Freud's place in this tradition in his obvious quest throughout his work to explore the correlations between the mind and the body. Along with the phenomenological theorists, Freud's work seemed to oppose the mind/body split espoused by Descartes in the seventeenth century.

In Chapter 3, I will begin with sociological perspectives on the body, including the work of Michel Foucault. My reason for using aspects of Foucault's work is to examine, with reference to psychiatric texts, how psychiatric discourse constructs mental illness in terms of its biological and bodily treatment and causation, to the neglect of what the patients' bodily presentation and appearance might express about their experiences. In this chapter, I provide a brief outline of the history of British psychiatry and the ways in which it has consistently focused upon the body and its observation. Interventions for depression and schizophrenia prevalent in the 1950s and 1960s, such as insulin therapy, epileptic shocks and ECT (electroconvulsive therapy), are all treatments aimed at affecting the body in order to treat the mind.

In Chapter 4, I discuss ways in which the body and mental illness have been approached within feminist theory. I first discuss socialist/Marxist feminist accounts of women's oppression as a whole. Although they say little about bodily expressions of mental illness, feminists such as Juliet Mitchell do identify how structural factors such as women's experiences of unemployment, their relation to the capitalist economy and their positions within the family are often influential in their oppression (these perspectives are still relevant today). These ideas have been applied to women's mental illness by sociologists such as Brown and Harris and Ann Oakley. These writers and others identify social factors as evoking mental illness in women. I state that these theorists say little about the body, but they do focus upon women's physical labour resulting from their roles as wives, mothers and carers. I proceed to discuss radical feminist thought that identifies patriarchy as responsible for women's oppression. I discuss how feminist writers, including Elaine Showalter, have identified psychiatry as a patriarchal system that serves to control the female body and sexuality.

In Chapter 5, I turn to psychoanalytic theory and the body in neurosis. I begin by providing a brief history of the construction and treatment of hysteria from the Greeks to Charcot. I then outline the work of Sigmund Freud and Joseph Breuer and their case studies of women patients suffering from hysteria. In a radical shift from previous accounts of hysteria, Freud and Breuer describe the body as communicating repressed psychical conflict and, in their treatment, attend to the language of the body in seeking to understand and treat the distress of their women patients.

I show how Freud's writings on the body consistently focus, as mentioned above, upon the correlation between psychical and physical processes and how these processes are essential to early development. His writings on infantile sexuality, for example, present the infant's body as a site of innumerable erotogenic zones through which the infant learns to relate to the outside world. In his writings of 1925 and beyond, Freud represents the needs of the female body as being psychically and physically motivated by a lack of a penis, with women's mental illness characterised by penis envy. Freud's admittedly rather sexist claims have provoked angry responses from feminist theorists including Kate Millett. However, in their focus upon Freud's sexism, feminist writers overall have tended to ignore his writings on the body.[4]

In Chapter 6, I discuss post-Freudian accounts on the body in psychosis. I begin by discussing the work of Paul Schilder who proposes that a person with psychosis lacks a sense of being in, or owning, their body due to a lack of libidinal investment in it. I then discuss the work of Jacques Lacan, whose writings, although challenging, are relevant to an understanding of the role of the body in the experience of psychosis.

Following my discussion of Lacan, I turn to the work of French feminist theorists Luce Irigaray and Julia Kristeva. I outline Irigaray's argument that the repression of female sexuality and language gives rise to women's mental illness. According to Irigaray, women's madness is manifested within their bodies. I also give an account of Kristeva's concept of the semiotic, which indicates the realm of the maternal body. She describes how women are closely bound with this realm to the extent that they are unable to enter the symbolic, which is referred to as the realm of language. Therefore, according to Kristeva, as Elizabeth Grosz states, women experience 'a fundamentally unspeakable experience, pleasure, or corporeality' (1990: 163).

I also focus upon Melanie Klein's concept that the infant's experience of complex internal objects through processes of projection and introjection, are valuable in the understanding of body image and psychosis in adults. I then examine the work of Wilfred Bion who discusses how in psychosis, the individual cannot tolerate frustration and will project out their feelings. He suggests that the psychotic person will respond to the world at the level of physical pleasure or pain and have reduced capacity for the tolerance that would enable thinking to bring about relief. I conclude this chapter with a discussion of R.D. Laing who describes how in psychosis, the person perceives a division between their sense of self and their body.

In Chapter 7, I propose that mental health practitioners might usefully pay attention to their own bodies when working with patients. Experiences including fear, tiredness, coldness and so on, may give us an indication of the experiences of the people we are caring for. I discuss the psycho-analytic concepts of transference, countertransference and body counter-transference. I discuss the point that Freud's understandings of transference were mostly in relation to people with neurosis. He stated that people with psychosis are unable to form a transference onto their analyst. However, this view was challenged following the work of Klein, who asserted that people with psychosis do appear to project feelings onto outside objects. I continue to develop Klein's view by discussing the work of post-Kleinians, including Herbert Rosenfeld and Margaret Little. I also discuss the concept of 'body countertransference' as discussed by Susie Orbach. The purpose of this chapter is to suggest that transference and both psychical and phys-ical countertransference feelings may be useful means of understanding interaction with, and the experiences of, people suffering mental illness. I state how I consider these concepts to place value and emphasis upon the lived experiences of people with mental illness.

The reader will no doubt notice that this book contains a significant amount of psychoanalysis. My intention is to demonstrate that psycho-analytic perspectives – although difficult and seemingly irrelevant – provide us with a confirmation that the 'symptoms' of people diagnosed with mental illness are meaningful. Freud (whose work is often seen to be irrelevant within large aspects of mental health practice) demonstrates his dedication to this notion in his early case studies on (mostly) female hysterics. As part of his 'Introductory Lectures on Psychoanalysis', in a paper entitled, 'Psycho-analysis and Psychiatry' (1917), Freud stated his criticism of psychiatry for not paying attention to the form and content of symptoms. In another paper, 'The sense of symptoms', he addresses how, in contrast to psychiatry, psychoanalysis asserts that a person's symptoms are mean-ingful and relate to their experiences. In other words, as Freud put it, symptoms 'have a connection with the life of those who produce them' (1917a: 258).

In Chapter 8, I detail my observations of two male and two female mental health patients. I provide a brief biographical background to each and discuss their diagnosis and treatment. The aim of this chapter is first to describe how these patients demonstrate their lived experience through their bodies and, second, to describe my psychical and physical responses to these expressions. I also outline my interactions with these patients and describe their accounts of their feelings about their bodies and the world around them. From my observations of these patients, their accounts of their experiences of their bodies and my psychical and physical counter-transference reactions to them, I offer an alternative 'reading' of the meanings apparent in their bodily presentation using the perspectives of embodiment from within sociology, feminism and psychoanalysis.

In Chapter 9, I draw together the issues raised in the book and suggest ways in which mental health practitioners can work with the body as communicator of lived experience within mental health practice. I empha-sise that mental health practitioners need to spend time thinking about, and being with, their patients in order to focus on their experiences. It is crucial they are supported in this process. In this chapter, I ask how possible insights into the experiences of patients might improve clinical practice.

This book is intended for mental health nurses, allied professionals and others with an interest in the body and mental illness. It is not intended to replace psychiatric practices but to add to current clinical understand-ings of the importance of the body in terms of its role in the experience of mental illness. I have carried with me my early fascination with the bodily presentations of people with mental illness. I hope to share this fascination with those who might read this book. I suggest that as mental health practitioners we can make room to think about our patients and what they might be communicating, often through bodily means, about their experiences in the world. This requires us to look beyond diagnosis at the person whose experiences are often very much alive and deserve recognition and respect.

# Chapter 2

# Lived experience

To understand the concept of 'lived experience' and the 'lived body', it is first necessary to define the meaning of phenomenology. This will be my starting point in this chapter, which will be followed by a brief outline of the work of the theorists Edmund Husserl and Maurice Merleau-Ponty in their understanding of experience and consciousness. The ideas of these phenomenological theorists basically opposed a philosophical and religious tradition that considered the body as inferior to the disembodied soul, mind and consciousness (as espoused by Descartes and often referred to as the 'mind/body split'). In contrast, Merleau-Ponty for example, positions the sensory and experiencing body 'before' the reflective consciousness. The action of thinking, itself, relates to the whole body. I shall state Freud's place in this tradition in his obvious dedication throughout his work to explore the correlations between the mind and the body. I will provide a further discussion of Freud's insights into the body and mental illness in Chapter 5.

## The mind/body split

The mind/body split actually has its origins in Greek philosophy. For the philosopher Plato (427–347 BCE), the 'matter' or physicality of the body is fundamentally inferior to the mind. The body is a threat to thought and reason, which rule over it. For Plato, the soul is linked to thought, which he states was created prior to the body. In *Timaeus*, Plato makes this clear: 'god created the soul before the body and gave it precedence both in time and value, and made it the dominating and controlling partner' (1977: 47). The body is presented by Plato as a kind of vessel or prison for the soul. The separation of the mind and body continued within the Christian tradition. The body was perceived as mortal. The immortal soul was derived from God, but also part of nature. René Descartes (1596–1650) was interested in the separation between the soul (the mind) and nature (the body).

## Cartesian dualism

Descartes proposed that the mind is a kind of thinking substance distinct from the body constituting nature. The mind refers to the soul and relates to consciousness. In *Meditations* (1641) he presents the world as mathematically describable and distinct from our sensory organs. This distinction became known as Cartesian dualism and it is this dualism that has greatly influenced the disciplines of science, medicine, ethics, morals and so on. Descartes is frequently described as responsible for laying the foundations of the 'modern' scientific age.

For someone so entrenched within a rational and scientific approach to life, Descartes' *Meditations* are rather poetic and moving. He writes about dreaming – is there anything to distinguish being asleep from being awake? Our unique judgements about the existence of things in the world are spurious and untrustworthy. The earth and the sky, colours and sounds could be the delusions of dreams; they do not confirm existence in themselves. It is thinking that ensures existence, *I am thinking, therefore I exist.* For Descartes, existence, thought and reason are God-given. In the third meditation, he refers to God as a craftsman, as a perfect being. A perfect idea cannot be merely thought up by the person thinking it; God has placed the idea there.[1]

Due to the influence of Cartesian dualism, 'reality' came to be seen as testable and measurable. The laws about how things work or exist can only be discerned by mathematical analysis. Phenomenologists stated that if we are reduced, as scientific inquiry suggests, to thinking about how things work or their existence, we miss out on our unique lived experience of them. Phenomenology opposed the sharp distinction between the mind and the body. Consciousness is not reduced to the mind and to thinking. It is located in the physical body, which is, according to Husserl, 'the medium of all perception; it is the organ of perception and is necessarily involved in all perception' (Husserl in Welton 1999: 12). Here Husserl is referring to his concept of the 'lived body'.

## Phenomenology

Phenomenology, then, is the study of consciousness as experienced from the first-person point of view. Often defined as the philosophy of experience, it focuses upon the structure of human experience including consciousness, imagination, desire, relations to others and embodied action (which was of particular concern to Merleau-Ponty as we shall see). Phenomenological research, therefore, advocates that there is no fixed, absolute reality. Reality is considered to only exist for the individual who perceives it. Subsequently, phenomenological research methods therefore focus upon individual experience and individual perception (Ramer cited in Nieswiadomy 1998: 151). Phenomenology can be considered in contrast to other philosophical disciplines such as ontology (the study of being), ethics (the study of right or wrong) or epistemology (the study of knowledge).

It supports three types of methods to explore consciousness. First, as human beings, we describe a type of experience as we perceive it in our experience. Second, we interpret our experiences by positioning them in or relating them to certain forms of context. Third, we analyse our experiences in order to make sense of them. Conscious experiences are unique in that we *experience* them and we *live* through them. We reflect upon our experiences after the event so to speak, but in order to do this we need to have a familiarity with our lived experiences. Consequently, Husserl and Merleau-Ponty described our capacity to provide a pure description of lived experience. It is this awareness or familiarity of lived experiences that enables the person to give a first-person account of the experience.

## Husserl and intentionality

The beginnings of phenomenology are marked by the work of Edmund Husserl (1859–1938). He was not opposed to the discipline of science in itself, but stated that it is important to acknowledge that it forms part of the same world in which we all have a common experience. He was interested in observations that do not just involve subjective experiences, but those that include attention to human relations within social networks (Weiss 1999: 39). For Husserl, a major component of the study of consciousness involves intentionality. Consciousness is always directed towards something.

In *Logical Investigations* (2001), Husserl outlined several aspects of philosophical thought ranging from logic to the philosophy of language, to a phenomenological theory of intentionality and a phenomenological theory of knowledge. Later in *Ideas Pertaining to a Pure Phenomenology and to a Phenomenological Philosophy* (in Welton 1999), he focused solely on phenomenology as the science of the essence of consciousness. Within this text, Husserl suggested a turning away from reality and a necessary move towards phenomena. He suggests that when we look at an object in the world we need not be concerned about whether it really exists. Our lived experience of something matters over whether something exists or not. If we reduce or bracket something in terms of its existence we lose interest in our experiences of it and, more specifically, the meaning or content that object has in terms of our individual experience.

## Merleau-Ponty: lived bodies

The work of Merleau-Ponty (1907–1961) developed Husserl's concept of the lived body. In the 1940s he developed a particular variation of phenomenology, which focused upon the role of the body in human experience.

Merleau-Ponty rejected intellectualist psychology, which focused upon the rational construction of the outside world in the mind. He states in *Phenomenology of Perception* (1945) that subjectivity is bound up with the body. The experience of being in the world is intrinsically tied to the experiences of being a body in the world. Merleau-Ponty's early work focused upon 'body image' particularly in relation to the experience of the amputee. The patient can still feel the pain in the limb that is no longer there. Traditional psychological understandings of this experience would suggest that the person is *remembering*. In this context the mind's cognitive abilities have a dominating role. The lost limb is somehow 'brought back' (through thinking) as if lost in the present situation. For Merleau-Ponty, the limb is *not* now absent, it is in fact present within the body image of the person. The person might well recognise that the limb is gone, but the actions or possibilities of the body remain. As Grosz puts it, the lost limb is 'quasi-present. It is the refusal of an experience to enter into the past; it illustrates the tenacity of a present that remains immutable' (1994: 89).

Stating his dedication to the relationship between the mind and the body, Merleau-Ponty suggests that the body's perceptiveness is not simply a result of what occurs in the realm of the mind. The mind itself is embodied. It is the body itself that 'learns' how to perform certain actions. As Merleau-Ponty states in *The Primacy of Perception*, 'a movement is learned when the body has understood it, that is, when it has incorporated it into its "world", and to move the body is to aim at things through it' (Merleau-Ponty in Welton 1999: 155). The body is a site of sensory experience, not a mere object. The mind is not separated from the body, or somehow just situated in the head with the body as a separate entity. Human beings perceive and experience the world through their bodies. Thought itself relates to the whole body in its relation to the world.

## Conclusion

I have briefly discussed the history of phenomenology, outlining the ideas of Husserl and Merleau-Ponty. These theorists offered an alternative to an understanding of consciousness as located purely in the realm of thinking. Merleau-Ponty applied these understandings to the body. These perspectives reveal that as human beings we are intrinsically, in bodily terms, linked to the world around us. Lived experiences refer to direct human experiences in the world. These experiences bring about certain responses and reactions in us: aching muscles, exhaustion, hazy and muddled feelings and emotions. It is as if the world responds to our emotions and at the same time demands responses and feelings from us. As Merleau-Ponty states, our bodies seem to directly relate to the objects around us even prior to us reflecting or conceptualising our actions. When we have dropped something, for example, it seems that our bodies automatically 'know' how to pick up the object without thinking about it.

Science attempts to define and quantify our actions. It is interested in measuring and quantifying the existence of things and how they function. Disorders of the mind are understood in terms of their cause in relation to chemical activity in the brain. The psychiatrist is interested in the frequency of mental distress. They will strive to assess the level of distress and the risk it poses to the sufferer and those around them in a measured manner. What is missed out is direct human experience. What led up to the 'disorder'? What happened in that person's life to bring about the 'symptom'?

A symptom, in my view, is a person's attempt to deal with their individual experiences of the world. An experience, if it cannot be tolerated, is swallowed down and seemingly forgotten. The experience is perhaps expelled outwards and the person creates a false reality to make living easier. In mental illness, then, the experience is perceived and communicated in an altered form, but of course it is still there. Merleau-Ponty offers a rather moving description of this process: 'we may overlook something although we know of it'. Our actions, which of course for Merleau-Ponty are bodily, display in general terms what has been repressed. Our experiences are not revealed in singular and conscious acts, but are, as Merleau-Ponty states, 'enveloped in generality. Through this generality we still "have them" but just enough to hold them at a distance from us' (ibid.: 162). We swallow things down to keep things with us, because we can't let go of them.

In a biomedical framework, we say the symptom does not mean anything and is just the result of chemical dysfunction. Symptoms are considered to relate to an illness that can be treated by medical interventions. How does a person with mental illness express his or her direct lived experience? I am suggesting that it is through symptoms that are often bodily. For Freud, a symptom is a consequence of an experience, a clue, or indication of it. He was interested in how experience was manifested. In his endeavour to find clues to the meanings inherent in symptoms, he focused upon the correlations between psychical and physiological processes, which remained with him throughout his work. His dedication to the links between the mind and body are apparent in his early work with hysterics. Experience is not expressed in words. It is unspoken. It is manifested in the body. In the next chapter, I will focus upon the body in terms of an 'outside-in' approach. The theorist Foucault suggested that outside prevailing discourses are inscribed upon the body. I will suggest how these ideas might be applied to an understanding of the *mentally ill* body.

# Chapter 3

# Bodily inscription

Explicit discussion of the body within sociology is a relatively recent development. As Chris Shilling points out in *The Body and Social Theory*, sociology has historically rarely focused upon the embodied human being 'as an object of importance in its own right' (1993: 19). The development of sociological discussion about the body has largely had as its focal point the work of Michel Foucault. As I stated in the Introduction, Foucault's writings are often difficult, but I hope to present them in a relevant and accessible manner here. Foucault's writings on the body can be understood as having two main components. First, an emphasis upon institutions that control and govern the body. Second, the assertion that the body is itself constructed through prevailing discourses. The purpose of this chapter is to apply Foucault's understanding of the body to mainstream mental health practice. I suggest that the mental health practitioner in their practice might consider how the *mentally ill body* is constructed by prevailing biomedical discourses and is subject to regulation by the institution of psychiatry. In other words, it is often the case that as practitioners we view the mentally ill person as a *biological subject.* I will then provide some brief examples of how, in Britain since the eighteenth century, mental illness has been understood and defined in relation to the body. I will then examine, with reference to psychiatric texts, and, considering my own background, nursing texts, the ways in which mainstream psychiatry focuses upon the body as a diagnostic index in the assessment process.

## Foucault: power, discourse and the body

An early formulation of the body by Foucault is evident in his essay 'Nietzsche, Genealogy, History'.[1] Here Foucault states that traditional approaches to history are dominated by assumptions that stem from certain notions of what people are like. Foucault states his disagreement with how history positions the 'reflective' and 'feeling' person as central. According to Foucault, essential human characteristics are wrongly considered to be necessary to the evolving of history.

Foucault asserts that historical events are normally understood to contain a true origin or essence and, subsequently, established knowledge is formulated and articulated in relation to such historical events. The following Nietzsche, Foucault presents, as a challenge to this way of thinking about history, the approach of the genealogist to historical events. The genealogist does not try to discover the first principles or origins of events that occur with the passage of time. In his book, *On the Genealogy of Morals*, for example, Nietzsche suggests with reference to genealogy, that events are subject to a series of 'ever-new interpretations and manipulations' (1996: 58), according to the particular circumstances in which they occur. Foucault focuses upon the role of the body rather than morals in the ways in which historical events are interpreted and shaped by prevailing constructs that alter and change.

Foucault states that the body does not merely have a physiological function that somehow escapes or remains neutral to outside constructs and practices unfolding throughout time. He suggests that such constructs and practices inscribe themselves onto the body, and genealogy serves to articulate this process:

> The body is the inscribed surface of events (traced by language and dissolved by ideas) . . . Genealogy, as an analysis of descent, is thus situated within the articulation of the body and history. Its task is to expose a body totally imprinted by history.
>
> (Foucault in Rabinow 1984: 83)

A frequently used literary reference to Foucault's body as an inscribed surface is Franz Kafka's *In the Penal Settlement* (or sometimes called the *Penal Colony*) written in 1919. An explorer has reluctantly, out of politeness, accepted the invitation by an officer to witness the execution of a soldier condemned to death because of disobedience. The officer explains to the explorer how an apparatus referred to as the Harrow will be used in the execution. The Harrow is made of glass so that its workings can be clearly observed from outside. It also has needles attached. The needles perform the task of writing upon the condemned man's body, beginning on his back and then on his front side. The Harrow continues to write for twelve hours. As is often the case with Kafka's work, there is no obvious 'meaning' or explanation apparent in this story. However, it seems to sum up, in a literary sense, Foucault's understanding of the body as inscribed by prevailing sets of beliefs.

For Foucault, history is a constant struggle between different power structures, which each attempt to impose their system of domination upon a given culture independent of human agency, or, in other words, the essential quality of humanness. Foucault suggests that power is not a group of structures, organisations or institutions operating from above. It does not refer to one group ruling or dominating another. He understands power as a system of negotiations *between* practices:

> I am not referring to Power – with a capital P – dominating and imposing its rationality upon the totality of the social body. In fact, there are power relations. They are multiple; they have different forms, they can be in play in family relations, or within an institution, or an administration.
>
> (Foucault in Jones and Porter 1994: 96)

The passive, pliable body is at the centre of the competition between different power structures for domination and an object upon which competing powers are negotiated. As Elizabeth Grosz asserts: 'The body is that materiality, almost a medium, on which power operates and through which it functions' (1994: 146). Power serves to produce an individual's desires for example, which, in turn, create certain knowledge about individuals. Subsequently, this knowledge produces improved and refined techniques for the surveillance of bodies. Therefore, the original power formation is reinforced and strengthened.

Foucault asserts that the body is also a focus of discourse and is the link between daily rituals and practices, and the larger structures of power. Shilling defines Foucault's use of the term discourse as: 'Sets of deep principles incorporating specific grids of meaning which underpin, generate and establish relations between all that can be seen, thought and said' (1993: 75). Discourses are constructed through the use of language and according to Foucault, as Bryan Turner summarises, 'it is only by language that we can know anything' (Turner 1984: 176).

The development of modernity, following the Enlightenment, influenced how discourses were formulated which directly influenced how individuals were constructed. This involved changes in the target, the object, and the scope of discourse. With regard to the target of discourse, the body as flesh was replaced by focus upon the mindful body, or rather the mind within the body. Alterations in the object of discourse brought about focus upon the structuring of life rather than concern with matters of death. Change in the scope of discourse brought about concern about the control of the differentiated population in a move away from the management of anonymous individuals. I will now outline three brief examples of Foucault's consideration of power and discourse and their effects upon the body and how these have changed over time. I will begin with *Madness and Civilisation* (1989), and then go on to discuss *Discipline and Punish* (1977) and *The History of Sexuality: Volume I* (1990).

Foucault first discusses the relationship between mental illness and medicine in *Mental Illness and Psychology*, which he wrote in 1954. In this work, Foucault outlines his critique of Freud, and presents mental illness as a social and cultural construct. He also describes how mental illness was generally accepted as a legitimate form of expression up to the beginning of the European Enlightenment in the middle of the seventeenth century. From this time onwards, according to Foucault, 'madness was to become the world of exclusion' (1954: 67). Those individuals showing signs of 'unreason' were confined within internment houses throughout Europe. Foucault develops this theme in *Madness and Civilisation* (1989), to which I will now turn.

## Foucault: *Madness and Civilisation*

In his chapter, 'The Great Confinement', Foucault asserts that internment houses contained the 'insane' as well as the unemployed, prisoners and the poor. Until the end of the eighteenth century, these individuals were confined within correction houses and the prevailing discourses articulated mental illness in terms of 'unreason' or as Foucault puts it, 'the scandal of unreason (1989: 81). Mental illness was thus considered as the lowest point of humanity.

At the beginning of the nineteenth century, the mentally ill were separated from prisoners and there was a move towards perceiving the mentally ill with benevolence. The outside chains upon the bodies of the mentally ill were banished. An example of this is evident in Foucault's much referenced depiction of Pinel removing the chains of the insane at Bicetre. Pinel responded to criticism of his action by asserting, 'I am convinced that these madmen are so intractable only because they have been deprived of air and liberty' (Pinel in Foucault, ibid.: 242). Foucault asserts that, although Pinel's actions were seen as liberating, they only served to identify the mentally ill as a new problem and consequently they were subjected to even more intensive, controlling confinement. Whereas mental illness was previously associated with unreason and absence of responsibility, it was now associated with morality. The emergence of the benevolent asylum, according to Foucault, was understood from the outside as indicative of liberation of the mentally ill and the ceasing of restraint. However, within the walls of the asylum the guilt of the mentally ill was organised by their keepers:

> The asylum no longer punished the madman's guilt, it is true; but it did more, it organised that guilt; it organized it for the madman as a consciousness of himself, and as a non-reciprocal relation to the keeper; it organised it for the man of reason as an awareness of the Other, a therapeutic intervention in the madman's existence.
>
> (ibid.: 247)

Foucault asserts that the bodies of the mentally ill were initially confined in a similar way to the criminal. Prevailing discourses about mental illness associated it with unreason, which, in turn, influenced how the mentally ill were treated. At the beginning of the nineteenth century with the introduction of the more benevolent asylum, the chains of the mentally ill were removed in an attempt to liberate them. Foucault then suggests the subsequent introduction of internal chains: the organisation of the guilt and moral responsibility of the mentally ill. By focusing upon these events, Foucault attempts to show how prevailing perceptions and discourses about the mentally ill served to produce knowledge that was used to further scrutinise, regulate and discipline their bodies.

## Foucault: *Discipline and Punish*

The transition away from the body as flesh toward the mindful body is evident in Foucault's *Discipline and Punish* (1977). Foucault's approach to history, which considers the body as inscribed by prevalent discourses that then produce knowledge that is used to further survey and control the body, forms the underlying principle in this work. Foucault outlines the ways in which modern institutions gain access to individuals and their bodies as well as their daily actions. He describes how, under monarchical law in the eighteenth century, punishment took place in public. The criminal's body was assaulted, torn apart and burned.

Foucault gives a gruesome account of the execution of Damiens the regicide in 1757 and the public execution of his body: 'The flesh will be torn from his breasts, arms, thighs and calves with red-hot pincers, his right hand, holding the knife with which he committed the said parricide, burnt with sulphur' (1977: 3). These descriptions suggest that the prisoner's body as flesh was publicly, and therefore visibly, condemned and tortured.

In contrast to public torture, Foucault presents an account of timetables of daily rituals imposed upon prisoners in Paris eighty years later. The prisoners are regulated by the clock, and in relation to their activities including rising, work, meals and so forth: 'At a quarter to six in the summer, a quarter to seven in winter, the prisoners go down into the courtyard where they must wash their hands and faces' and 'After the dinner, there is recreation until twenty minutes to eleven' (ibid.: 6). Foucault describes the disappearance of the torture of bodies as a public spectacle, which was replaced by institutional regulations. The outside of the body is no longer punished and there is no longer a visible show of punishment. A hold upon the body ceased and was replaced by control and regulation of prisoners' minds.

In relation to these ideas, Shilling points out that those who governed prison systems of the nineteenth century, 'scientifically managed institutional space' (1993: 76) so as to gain access to prisoners' minds. This process was epitomised by a prison design created by Jeremy Bentham and referred to as the Panopticon. According to Foucault, in this system prisoners were surveyed constantly under the gaze of those who governed them. They were under surveillance by the Panopticon, a central tower, and subsequently pressured to manage and control their own behaviour. The model of the Panopticon moved into other social institutions including schools, army barracks and hospitals. There was, therefore, a shift in the scope of discourse. This was located in the move away from the control of individual bodies to the regulation of the social body.

## Foucault: *The History of Sexuality*

Foucault also asserts in his analysis of sexuality, that the body was similarly transformed in this context. The arena where sexuality was articulated in the Middle Ages was within the Christian confession. There was concern among priests with the bodily activity of sex and thus discourses about sex focused upon the body as flesh. The Reformation and the Counter-Reformation introduced a focus upon the individual's conscious intentions and action. Thus, the focus of sexuality moved away from the body and was replaced by discourse that served to discipline and control the mind. These discourses were reinforced by outside governing forces and contained within the mind of the individual. In *The History of Sexuality: Volume 1* Foucault states that this transition can be located within a number of institutions and disciplines including medicine, psychiatry, biology and psychology.

## Criticisms of Foucault

By focusing upon psychiatry, prison systems and sexuality, Foucault reveals the processes by which dominant discourses are formulated and serve to create further ways to manage and discipline groups of individuals. The texts I have outlined have attracted much criticism from historians. Felix Driver outlines some criticisms towards Foucault's *Discipline and Punish*. Historians, according to Driver, have questioned whether the transition between punitive regimes was as clear-cut as Foucault asserts. Foucault's critics also question whether there existed differing practices within different institutions, or whether there were conflicts between prisoners and those who governed them. However, Driver states that Foucault has attempted to answer these questions and defended his account of prison systems. In these discussions, Foucault clearly aims to outline how disciplinary strategies have emerged and impacted upon prison systems, rather than to 'reconstruct the history of the prison system in all its complexity' (Driver in Jones and Porter 1994: 119).

Turner in *The Body and Society* (1984) states that Foucault tends to consider that discourse has universal social consequences. Turner gives the example of confessional discourse in medieval times. According to a

Foucauldian perspective, all individuals, irrespective of their class or gender, have conducted confessions in a similar way. Turner argues in response to this that it is almost impossible to understand discourse outside the social context in which it is formed. Turner also asserts that what is absent in Foucault's account of discourse is any acknowledgement of the different social groups which are the 'targets and bearers' (1984: 175) of discourse.

The concept of the body as the focus of discourse has also received criticism. Bodies, in Foucauldian terms, are contained within disciplinary practices and systems. He says little about the body as the individual lives it. Turner states that although Foucault discusses pleasure and desire in some detail, he does not acknowledge the sensual bodily experiences of individuals. As people, we have a unique, personalised relationship to our bodies. We occupy our own bodies. Foucault emphasises instead that outside agencies control and have ownership of our bodies. In the case of medicine, for example, in Foucauldian terms, experts hold knowledge about how the body functions, and its needs.

With reference to his concept of the body, Foucault has also been referred to as 'gender-blind'. Sandra Lee Bartky states that Foucault's analysis of the body and power tends to neglect how techniques disciplining the body are frequently gendered. Bartky analyses how the female body is controlled and disciplined within a regime she refers to as the 'disciplinary regime of femininity'. She states how Foucault is blind to these disciplines and appears to consider that the female body has no determinate quality that is distinct from the male norm. Foucault, according to Bartky, approaches the body 'as if bodily experiences of men and women did not differ' (Bartky in Diamond and Quinby 1988: 63).

As I have stated, Foucault's work has provoked much criticism from historians with regard to the accuracy of his account of historical events. In addition, Foucault has been accused of gender-blindness and for not paying attention to the individual's lived, sensual experience of their body. According to Foucault, a person cannot experience an authentic emotion. For instance, when we look at something beautiful and feel moved, we tend to think that the feeling – which we often cannot put into words – is something essentially human. We often think that we are born with the capacity for these feelings. According to Foucault, such experiences are shaped and informed by prevailing discourses. Somewhere along the way we have internalised the knowledge that sunsets or a bright night sky are beautiful. In this context, Foucault can be considered as anti-humanistic. However, despite these criticisms, Foucault's work is useful in understanding the effects of discourse and power on the body. It is my intention to apply Foucault's concepts to an understanding of mental illness and the body. In this context, the *mentally ill* body is inscribed by popular discourses about mental illness. The prevailing discourses existing within mental health practice, as we will now see, consider the cause of mental illness to stem from biomedical factors such as brain chemical dysfunction. These approaches consequently influence how we view the bodies of those with mental illness.

I will now provide a brief discussion of how mental illness has been understood and defined in Britain. The so-called therapeutic interventions for depression and schizophrenia prevalent in the 1950s and 1960s – such as insulin therapy, epileptic shocks and ECT – all involved the treatment of the body in order to treat the mind. I will then go on to discuss modern mental health practice. As we shall see, prevailing discourses currently consider the causes of mental illness as stemming from biomedical factors including biochemical brain dysfunction. My intention is to explore whether psychiatry acknowledges an understanding of embodiment from other disciplines, which explore how individuals express their lived experience through their bodies, as well as the biological symptoms of their mental illness.

## The beginnings of psychiatry

Throughout history, mental illness or madness has been formulated using a radically different range of concepts. Early Greek concepts considered it as a consequence of divine or demonic possession (I will discuss this in more detail in Chapter 5). Christian and medieval Islamic medicine advocated an understanding of mental illness from Hippocratic medicine. Mental illness in this context was understood, not in terms of the influence of gods and demons, but in terms of the 'fluids' or 'humours' of the body. These consisted of blood, yellow bile, phlegm and melancholy. An individual with an excess of blood for example, would be considered as susceptible to outbursts of temper and mania. A body with an excess of black bile was considered as prone to depression and so forth. This view was challenged by the increasing influence of medicine and science taking place in the eighteenth century. According to Edward Shorter (1997), this marked the introduction of naturalistic and rational concepts of mental illness. This 'new science' placed emphasis upon the solids – nerves, fibres and organs – of the body.

Focus upon the solids of the body, which arose with the rise of scientific medicine, suggested that the cause of mental illness had as its foundation the lesions of the body that was considered to consist of a system of electrical piping, which connected the limbs to the brain. This viewpoint, according to Roy Porter (2002), reinforced the Cartesian notion of a mind/body split. The soul came to be seen as incapable of being violated, and the body and its workings were seen to cause mental illness. Porter cites as an example of this emphasis upon the body, the work of a London physician Thomas Willis (1621–1675) who coined the term 'neurology'. Willis stated that the nervous system was influenced by, as Porter describes, 'the operations of animal spirits, superfine chemical intermediaries between body and mind capable of being affected by either' (2002: 124). Similarly, a colleague of Willis, Richard Mead, argued that the false ideas experienced by the mentally ill were caused by disordered animal spirits that manifested themselves in the limbs causing uncontrolled movements. Porter also cites the work of Nicholas Robinson who, in *A New System of the Spleen* in 1729, stated that changes in bodily organs consequently caused changes in the mind.

## Neurology

These ideas set the scene for what Shorter refers to as the 'first biological psychiatry', in the nineteenth century, which focused upon how the brain and its structures were possibly responsible for the onset of mental illness. The scientific investigation into mental illness, which was dominated by German physicians in the nineteenth century, took place within universities and institutes as part of a wider interest in medical research. As Shorter states: 'Doctors began to apply the clinical-pathological method: reasoning back and forth from findings at autopsy to the signs and symptoms the patient displayed before death' (1997: 70).

One German physician within this period was Theodor Meynert, who placed emphasis upon anatomy in the understanding of the onset of mental illness. He focused particularly upon the microscopic structure of the brain and distinguishing certain layers and other particular parts. He published his first textbook in 1884 in which he describes in careful detail the brain and, in particular, the workings of the frontal lobes, which were to be considered as particularly relevant to the onset of mental illness. Shorter describes this text as a 'manual of neuroanatomy, punctured with hypothetical observations about the frontal lobes as the inhibitory centers and the subcortical regions as the stimulative ones' (ibid.: 347). Another physician in this area of research was Paul Flechsig, who also studied neuroanatomy. He was significant in being responsible for the development of cerebral localisation, detailing how different locations of the brain were responsible for different functions.

The perspectives I have outlined focus upon bodily and neurological factors as causes of the symptoms of mental illness in the context of increased scientific investigation into both medical and mental illness. I will now turn to physical interventions and therapies that have been used to treat mental illness, specifically insulin coma and ECT.

## Physical interventions

The treatment of insulin coma therapy has its foundations in the procedure of treating mental illness with prolonged sleep. A young physician,

Neil Macleod, in 1897, administered a woman with psychosis a large dose of bromide. She was suffering from 'nervous shock' following news of a family crisis and subsequently developed mania. After receiving a large dose of bromide and after a long sleep lasting several days, she recovered from her mental distress. This procedure was developed within psychiatric practice, and the drug bromide was replaced by barbiturates, in particular barbital.

The hormone insulin had been given to patients in the 1920s to increase their appetites when they refused to eat. Manfred Sakel in 1933 first introduced it in Austria as a curative procedure for mentally ill patients. He first gave insulin to people addicted to morphine and found that it curtailed their desire for it. He then discovered that putting mentally ill patients, in particular those suffering from schizophrenia, into an insulin coma appeared to alleviate their symptoms. The coma resulted from the insulin causing the patient's blood sugar to drop to very low levels. The patient would remain in a coma for twenty minutes and was then brought back to consciousness with glucose administered directly into the stomach. This procedure has been widely used in Britain and the US. Shorter reports, for example, that by the 1960s in America, there were insulin units in over a hundred hospitals (1997: 212).

Following on from the introduction of insulin in the treatment of mental illness, patients began to be treated with 'convulsive therapy', whereby epileptic fits were produced by the administration of a drug named Cardiazol (known as Metrazol in the US). In 1929, a neuropathologist named Ladislas von Meduna, reported as a result of carrying out autopsies on epileptic patients, that their brains were different in structure to those with schizophrenia. At this time, it was also reported that epileptic patients who developed schizophrenia, suffered less frequently from epileptic fits. Meduna began to consider the reverse, whether or not the symptoms of schizophrenia improved with the development of epileptic fits. The result was that many patients improved by this method, although the drug Cardiazol produced many side effects including vomiting, pain in the muscles, and anxiety prior to the onset of the fit. This medication also caused patients, as a result of their fits, to sustain broken bones.

The physical procedure that followed on from Cardiazol administration was ECT. This was introduced by Ugo Cerletti in 1938, and is still used today surrounded by much controversy. There is no clear explanation of how ECT actually works and there are concerns about the side effects of this treatment. The procedure is carried out by producing electric convulsions in the patient by placing two electrodes on each side of the head. Cerletti and his colleagues found that this procedure could alleviate the symptoms of schizophrenia and, particularly, severe depression. ECT is thought to be more successful than 'convulsive therapy' because it causes fewer side effects than the administration of Cardiazol. The physical therapies of insulin coma and ECT brought about a radical shift within psychiatric thought away from the dominance of neurology. Such physical therapies also included the introduction of pharmacological therapies for the treatment of mental illness.

## Pharmacological treatments

Pharmacological therapies have been used within psychiatric practice since the Middle Ages. Laxatives, for example, were a very common treatment that supported the hypothesis that dangerous toxins influencing the mind gathered in the colon and needed to be expelled. This treatment for 'insanity' continued to be used into the twentieth century. In the 1920s for example, English psychiatrists still supported this practice by administrating croton oil, which induces diarrhoea, to curtail a mental crisis.

The introduction of anti-psychotic medication in the 1950s was a turning point for psychiatry. Patients who were previously considered as uncontrollable could now be managed more effectively. For the management of schizophrenia, the drug Chlorpromazine was introduced in 1953. In America, Chlorpromazine and other drugs of its type became referred to as 'anti-psychotic' medication. The effects of these medications, which also include thioridazine and trifluoperazine, act by controlling over-active, disturbed behaviour and agitation. They have a general depressant action on the central nervous system, but their main action is on the subcortical structures of the brain. These include the limbic system, which is concerned with emotional reactions; the hypothalamus, which is concerned with the autonomic centres; and the reticular system that is responsible for producing and maintaining a state of awareness.

More recently, during the 1980s, there has been the introduction of the 'dopamine hypothesis'. It is thought that patients with schizophrenia produce an excess of dopamine in their brains. This hypothesis is supported by research that shows that administration of dopaminergic agents can cause psychotic behaviour. Research suggests that some anti-psychotic drugs act by binding dopamine sites, thereby reducing psychotic symptoms. In depression, it is thought that there is a decrease in the brain chemicals serotonin and noradrenaline. Anti-depressant medication such as MAOIs (monoamine oxidase inhibitors) among them phenelzine, and SSRIs (selective serotonin reuptake inhibitors) including fluvoxamine and fluoxetine, act by increasing these brain chemicals.

## Contemporary psychiatry

I have provided some brief examples of how psychiatry has focused upon bodily and biological causes and interventions for the treatment of mental illness. I will now examine contemporary psychiatric texts and aim to explore what they say about the body and embodiment in terms of the presentation of mental illness.

One of the principal roles of the psychiatrist is to diagnose a patient who appears to be suffering from psychiatric symptoms and to formulate an effective treatment. A patient suffering from schizophrenia, for example, the most common psychotic disorder, is likely to exhibit symptoms relating to abnormalities in perception, beliefs, thought processes and expression. The schizophrenic may experience second- and third-person 'auditory hallucinations', 'delusional beliefs' and 'ideas of reference' whereby they may believe that something on the media or on television intrinsically relates to them. They may suffer from 'thought insertion' believing that their thoughts and bodily functions are under external control. 'Negative symptoms' include blunting of affect and emotion – many patients suffering from 'schizophrenia' find it difficult to get the meaning of an ironic joke, or to 'read between the lines' in another's speech. Other so-called 'negative' symptoms include apathy, self-neglect and social withdrawal.

Two strands of thought would be likely to influence a psychiatrist formulating a diagnosis of a patient with schizophrenia. First and foremost they would consider a biomedical approach. They may consider recent developments in neuroimaging that have tentatively identified certain functional and structural abnormalities in the brain as a cause of schizophrenia. The dominant approach to schizophrenia is one that is neuropharmacological. As I have stated above, it is considered that the brain of these patients produces too much dopamine. The treatment will consequently consist of medication that serves to block the release of dopamine and other receptors in the brain. Genetic explanations are also considered. Twin and family studies are also indicated as evidence of genetic causes of schizophrenia. Other factors, such as obstetric complications and birth and pregnancy difficulties in the mothers of schizophrenic patients, are also frequently listed as causative factors.

## Psychiatric textbooks

I will now examine two psychiatric texts. I will consider the *International Classification of Diseases (ICD-10)*,[2] which is a collaborative text produced by the World Health Organisation and intended for use by psychiatrists as a diagnostic manual. Using a numerical framework, the *ICD-10* categorises mental and behavioural disorders according to various symptoms. Second, I will review the *Shorter Oxford Textbook of Psychiatry* (2001), which is a standard text used in the training of psychiatrists and a reference book for practising psychiatrists. In my focus upon these texts, I will consider what they say about the body in relation to mental illness.

With regards to reference to the body and the bodily presentation and appearance of patients with mental illness, the *ICD-10* states how the symptoms of conditions such as schizophrenia can bring about a reduced ability to care for physical appearance. The list of symptoms provided for the diagnosing of schizophrenia, include among bodily presentations, the phrase 'poor social performance or self-care' (WHO 1993: 68).

The body is mentioned in *ICD-10*'s account of the symptoms of conditions such as 'schizophrenia', 'depressive disorder', 'dissociative disorder' and 'somatoform disorder'. Schizophrenia, for example, is described as producing hallucinations that may be in the form of voices giving a commentary on the affected person's behaviour, or 'other types of hallucinatory voices coming from some part of the body' (ibid.: 64). In the case of paranoid schizophrenia, the individual is considered to experience delusions that consist of 'bodily change, hallucinations of smell or taste, sexual or other bodily sensations' (ibid.: 66). Severe depression is described as producing possible delusions of worthlessness or bodily disease. *ICD-10* describes dissociative disorders as the contemporary term for hysteria. It is stated that the individual will complain of physical symptoms which upon clinical investigation have no medical basis, but have a psychological cause: 'There is a persistent severe and distressing pain in any part of the body, which cannot be explained adequately by evidence of a physiological process or a physical disorder' (ibid.: 108).

Dissociative disorder is described as relating to past traumatic events and the sufferer will exhibit symptoms that represent the patient's own concept of how physical illness would appear. The *ICD-10* does acknowledge that dissociative disorder is an expression of emotional needs and conflicts. Somatoform disorder describes the presentation of physical symptoms and the persistent requests for medical investigation of these, even after reassurance has been given about the absence of a medical condition.

*ICD-10* thus categorises how the body can manifest symptoms that indicate the psychological experiences of the patient. This may invite the lay reader to consider how the body is an important tool through which an individual can communicate their mental distress. However, the manual does not stress this point. Bodily manifestations are primarily described as the basis by which psychiatric diagnoses of dissociative disorder or somatoform disorder can be made and appropriate treatment given. This manual does not emphasise how the body may express the experiences of the individual other than the symptoms that relate to their psychiatric diagnosis.

The *Shorter Oxford Textbook of Psychiatry* discusses the body in terms of disorders of eating including anorexia and bulimia. The textbook acknowledges that such eating difficulties are predominantly experienced by women, and suggests that it is first necessary for psychiatrists, when assessing such patients, to assess the patient's physical state and to identify cases that might benefit from anti-depressant medication. The textbook suggests that eating difficulties stem predominantly from biological or behavioural problems, and behavioural therapies can help normalise eating patterns.

Obesity is considered in the *Shorter Oxford Textbook of Psychiatry* as stemming predominantly from genetic factors that are then exacerbated by social factors that encourage individuals to overeat. Sex differences are not explored in relation to obesity. Similarly, psychological factors do not seem to be considered: 'psychological causes do not seem to be of great importance in most cases' (Gelder *et al.* 2001: 454). The textbook does consider 'binge eating disorder' as manifesting itself alongside decreased self-esteem and social confidence. However, the textbook concludes its consideration of 'binge eating disorder' by stating that overweight people in general show no more psychological disturbance than the general population. Suggestions for treatment indicate that 'mildly' overweight people require merely good advice about diet and exercise. For obese individuals the prognosis is grim: 'Long-term results of all kinds of treatments are disappointing whether supervised by a doctor or not' (ibid.: 455). These treatments include self-help groups, appetite suppressants and behavioural treatments. The textbook indicates that eating difficulties stem overall from biological, behavioural and genetic factors.

Attention to patients' bodily presentation and appearance is emphasised within the textbook in its discussion of assessments. These take place when a patient is first admitted to hospital and include assessment of the patient's mental state. It is suggested that the psychiatrist observes the general appearance of the patient so as to identify psychiatric and psychological conditions including 'self-neglect', 'alcoholism', 'drug addition', 'dementia', 'depression' and 'schizophrenia'. Focus upon body build is emphasised to observe possible signs of 'anorexia', 'depression' or 'chronic anxiety states', which may, for example, have caused recent weight loss. Facial expression is specified; a depressed person may turn down the corners of their mouth or have vertical furrows on their brow. The textbook states that an anxious patient may have horizontal creases on their forehead. The depressed patient is also described as likely to lean forward with shoulders hunched, the head inclined downwards, and their gaze directed to the floor. An anxious patient is described as likely to frequently touch their jewellery, adjust their clothing and pick at their fingernails (ibid.: 42).

There is much emphasis upon observation of the body during an assessment to identify possible psychiatric conditions. Thus, it can be considered that a patient's physical appearance may be used as a diagnostic index, as the textbook suggests: 'Much can be learnt from the patient's appearance and behaviour. The patient's *general appearance* repays careful observation. A dirty unkempt look and crumpled clothing may indicate self-neglect' (ibid.). As well as making an initial assessment that involves observation of the patient's mental and physical state, psychiatrists are advised to observe patients within their ongoing interactions with them.

Emphasis upon body and dress during the assessment process is also considered in relation to 'depressive disorders' and 'mania'. The depressed patient is considered as likely to neglect dress and grooming. The manic patient's appearance is seen as congruous with mood that is often elated: 'Manic patients may wear bright colours, or dress incongruously' (ibid.). Oddity of dress is also described as a clue to schizophrenia. The textbook clearly states that an untidy or inappropriate appearance reflects an unhealthy mental state that begs a diagnostic definition. A clean tidy appearance is described as appropriate and is considered as congruent with good mental health.

Descriptions of symptoms of various forms of mental illness are made in the textbook using a universal 'he'. An exception to this can be found when the textbook suggests how odd clothing may be a clue to the thoughts of the individual: 'a rain-hood worn on a dry day may be the first evidence of a patient's belief that rays are being shone on her head' (ibid.). Leaving aside the possibility of incomplete editing, it is not clear why the textbook has switched to using a female pronoun. It could indicate value judgements suggesting that oddity in clothing is less acceptable in women. Reference to women patients can also be found within discussions of schizophrenic conditions in relation to dress sense: 'Self care may be poor and, particularly in women, the style of dress and presentation may be careful but somewhat inappropriate' (ibid.: 333).

The *Shorter Oxford Textbook of Psychiatry* does indicate that certain clinical features associated with conditions such as schizophrenia and dissociative disorders include specific bodily aspects. Schizophrenia is described as either acute or chronic. Bodily manifestations are described in relation to the chronic form. 'Waxy flexibility' for example, is cited as a chronic symptom involving the patient remaining in an 'awkward posture for longer than most people could achieve without discomfort' (ibid.). These postures are also considered to have a symbolic significance, such as that of crucifixion. This may indicate that the patient has a delusional schizophrenic belief that he is Christ. The textbook also specifies how an individual with schizophrenia may exhibit motor symptoms and signs including tics, unusual movements such as rocking to and fro, and grimacing. There are also physical signs described such as echopraxia where the patient will imitate the movements of the interviewer.

The textbook does explore how in some psychiatric disorders there are disorders within the body image. These include believing a limb to be still there following amputation or an incorrect belief that a limb is missing. The textbook discusses the distortion in body image in anorexia. The distorted awareness of the size and shape of the body, such as the feeling that a limb is enlarging, is discussed in relation to epilepsy and drug use, in particular LSD. The textbook describes how in schizophrenia, there sometimes occurs a 'reduplication phenomenon' whereby the sufferer will believe that their body, or part of their body, has doubled. 'Body dysmorphic disorder' is described as a concern by the sufferer that part of their body is misshapen or distorted. There is no discussion of the possible causes of these conditions or the implications for the subjective experience of the individual involved.

'Somatoform disorder' and 'dissociative' or 'conversion disorder' are recognised as a presentation of symptoms stemming from a psychological cause. The physical symptoms apparent in these conditions may include 'paralysis of a limb', 'impaired coordination', 'aphonia', 'mutism', and sensory symptoms such as deafness and blindness. The textbook suggests that many patients are reluctant to accept that their bodily symptoms have a psychological basis. The textbook discusses the various explanations for these conditions. Cultural factors are discussed whereby in non-Western settings these disorders may be considered as possession states. There is also research cited that points to neuroimaging and biological techniques that specify that these disorders may be the result of abnormalities in brain function. Psychodynamic theories are described briefly as making use 'of the concept of conversion of distress into physical symptoms having symbolic meaning' (ibid.: 255).

Suggested treatments include behavioural techniques such as anxiety management and cognitive therapy with an intention to move emphasis away from the symptoms and to focus upon the factors that provoked the disorder. The textbook describes how the patient should be informed that their symptoms are caused by psychological factors and not physical disease. Furthermore, the patient should be informed that, 'if they try hard to regain control, they will succeed' (ibid.: 256).

## Summary of psychiatric texts

In the discussion of the body and embodiment, both the *ICD-10* and *Shorter Oxford Textbook of Psychiatry*, refer to the psychiatric conditions 'self-harm', 'disorders of eating', 'schizophrenia', 'mania', 'depressive disorders', 'dissociative disorder' and 'somatoform disorder'. The textbooks appear to emphasise the behavioural aspects of these conditions with a view to normalising behaviour. It is also stated that these conditions have a biological and genetic basis. It is only 'dissociative' and 'somatoform disorder' that are described as having a psychological basis that is expressed through bodily means. In the discussion of the physical appearance of patients, the textbooks offer no analysis of bodily presentation and appearance other than stating that 'inappropriate' self-care and dress indicate a possible psychiatric condition such as depressive disorder or schizophrenia, which requires clinical treatment. Additionally, the textbooks do not clarify what 'inappropriate' actually refers to and with regard to whom. References to women patients that are presented as a clear shift away from the universal 'he' and stated within discussions about oddity of clothing, possibly reflect how society considers that the inappropriate appearance and demeanour of women is less acceptable than that of men. Furthermore, the textbooks make little reference to cultural values about mental illness and how the bodies of people with mental illness and the way we see them can reflect prevailing discourses about mental illness and its presentation. The textbook emphasises the importance of observing the body, but only as an indicator of possible psychiatric conditions. Therefore, the body in psychiatry is a site containing clues to psychiatric diagnosis. The body does not hold clues to the emotional experience of the individual, and how patients have made sense of themselves and the world around them.

## Mental health nursing

The radical psychiatrist Peter Breggin in *Toxic Psychiatry* (1993) describes a hierarchical pyramid whereby the psychiatrist is positioned at the top and the *female* patient is at the very bottom (1993: 402). In terms of status and influence, nurses are positioned below psychiatrists in the mental health hierarchy at a level congruous with ancillary professionals including social workers and occupational therapists. Nurses have more interaction with patients than psychiatrists or perhaps any other professional, and are responsible for implementing individual patient care plans under the supervision of a psychiatrist, which involve an assessment of individual patient needs, and goals to be achieved. The nurse will be responsible for the care of patients along with other members of the multi-disciplinary team. However, the prime responsibility for patients in terms of diagnosis, treatment and discharge lies in the hands of the psychiatrist, as Joan Busfield points out, using a Foucauldian understanding of discourse, 'psychiatrists formally construct the dominant social discourse through which mental disorder is constituted and given meaning' (1996: 51).

## Nursing textbooks

The first mental health nursing textbook (textbook A) considered will be *A Textbook of Psychiatric and Mental Health Nursing*.[3] This textbook was written specifically for the 'Project 2000: A New Preparation for Practice' training course set up in 1986. This course aimed to provide nurses with 'a generic preparation before specialisation' (Brooking *et al.* 1992: 39), which involves a multi-disciplinary approach to practice. *A Textbook of Psychiatric and Mental Health Nursing* was identified as a major textbook for the Project 2000 course and as a source of reference for qualified nurses. The second textbook (B) will be *Lyttle's Mental Health and Disorder* (Thompson and Mathias 2000), which is also used widely by pre-registration mental health nurses. In the examination of these textbooks the following issues will be considered: What do the texts say about the body in relation to mental illness? Do the texts consider whether patients may express their emotional and cultural experience through their bodily presentation and appearance?

When reviewing the texts for references to the body and mental illness, I observed how they usefully discuss sex differences in relation to the presentation of mental illness and to psychiatric diagnosis. I have chosen to outline these factors as I feel they relate to the case studies I present in Chapter 8, where I describe two men and two women. It appears that men and women present their distress differently and different factors contribute to their mental illness. I discuss these factors in more detail in Chapter 8, and for now will briefly outline the focus upon sex differences in this nursing text.

Textbook A points out that men are most likely to be diagnosed with conditions such as 'alcoholism' and 'schizophrenia' during their twenties and women are more likely to be diagnosed with 'neurotic' disorders including depression and anxiety. According to this textbook, women's social position also appears to relate to patterns of psychiatric diagnosis. It reports that women who are married and those with young children are more frequently diagnosed with mental illness. Social class is also identified as a contributory factor influencing psychiatric diagnosis. Working-class women are identified as being more likely to experience depression than middle-class women. Additionally, they are more likely to experience job loss, financial difficulties, marital breakdown, larger families and poor housing. The textbook identifies these factors as contributing to the onset of mental illness, especially depression. These factors are considered to increase a woman's vulnerability and significantly reduce her self-esteem.

Twice as many women than men are seen as likely to self-harm, which is characterised by acts such as cutting and self-poisoning. Textbook B, however, describes how this gender gap has closed over recent years. In addition, suicidal behaviour used to be associated with men over seventy-five, but it now appears that greater numbers of young men successfully kill themselves (Thompson and Mathias 2000: 390).

The textbooks discuss how gender role stereotyping may provide some explanation of such differences. Due to the effects of socialisation, stereotypical male roles are perceived as being emotionally restrained and self-sufficient, whereas female roles are seen as more help seeking and emotionally based. Textbook A suggests that as a consequence of this, women rather than men, 'are more likely to see their problems as a type of mental disorder and are more likely to seek psychiatric help for them' (Brooking et al. 1992: 149). Additionally, the textbook states that such differences may be due to the ways in which psychiatrists are influenced by gender role stereotyping, and suggests that it is likely that sex differences in relation to diagnosis are 'at least in part the result of professional patterns of gender-based diagnosis' (ibid.). However, the textbook does not elaborate on this point and claims that, although there is some evidence to support this hypothesis, 'there is no systematic picture of how this works' (ibid.). Textbook B suggests that the female role in society is more closely related to the sick role and this explains why women are more frequently diagnosed with depression and other 'neurotic' disorders. For a woman to be depressed is more socially acceptable than a man expressing similar complaints (Thompson and Mathias 2000: 378).

Textbook A discusses various studies involving gender role stereotyping and the social values attached to women and men's roles. These values are shown to relate to the ways in which men and women are seen in relation to their mental health. For example, the text outlines a 1970 study by Broverman *et al.*, which involved a group of mental health practitioners asked to consider the characteristics that constitute a 'mentally healthy man', 'a mentally healthy woman' and a 'mentally healthy adult independent of sex'. The findings of the study reported that the characteristics of a mentally healthy adult independent of sex were found to match those of a mentally healthy man, but not those of a healthy woman.

Other research is discussed which indicates how doctors may be influenced by stereotypes of femininity within medicine. Doctors have been shown to diagnose women as having psychological disorders when their symptoms may, in fact, be physically caused. For example, women reporting dysmenorrhoea or infant colic are often labelled as 'neurotic'. Similarly, women recovering from hysterectomy are perceived by doctors as automatically likely to suffer from grief following the loss of their reproductive functions. The textbook describes a 1987 study by Webb, which has confirmed that women's low feelings are more likely to be associated with post-operative infections. The textbook acknowledges that gender role stereotyping may be prevalent among psychiatrists, psychologists and psychotherapists due to their being reared in a sexist culture that places women into particular roles and influenced by the process of socialisation. Mental health nurses are also considered as likely to be influenced by gender stereotypes in their clinical practice with patients.

The textbook goes some way towards reflecting the now widely accepted feminist view linking women's mental distress with popularly held stereotypes about women's proper role. The women's movement in the past two decades has emphasised the importance of women's mental health issues in a societal context. The textbook refers to Phyllis Chesler's *Women and Madness* (1997), for example, which considers how women's mental distress can result from gender role stereotyping. Chesler describes how women's rejection of such roles leads to them being labelled as sick or psychologically deviant. The textbook, however, appears to be tentative in its criticism of psychiatry and its treatment of women. It introduces a sociological perspective in its discussion of social factors contributing to women's mental distress and the effects of socialisation, but does not provide a wider cultural critique such as that found within feminist discourse.

With regard to any discussion about bodily presentation and appearance, Textbook A presents a similar picture to the *ICD-10* reviewed above. Bodily presentation is discussed in relation to 'depression', 'mania', 'schizophrenia', 'eating disorders' and 'dissociative disorder'. Dissociative disorder is the only condition that is not considered as having a biological cause. The patient is stated as presenting physical symptoms such as paralysis of a limb, which stems from a psychological, not medical, cause.

Textbook B, within its discussion of mental health problems, discusses certain psychiatric conditions that involve the body or somatic health. 'Hypochrondriasis' involves a patient believing that they are physically unwell when they are not, and where several areas of the body may be involved. It is noted that such patients may be depressed and present themselves as fragile. They are difficult to reassure and may seek the advice of several different doctors in an attempt to have their complaints taken seriously. 'Malingering' is described as a condition where the sufferer will fabricate certain health problems or where there is an exaggerated emphasis upon health problems. The textbook suggests that these two conditions are not clearly attributed to mental illness, but may 'be seen to form the parameters of somatic health related problems' (Thompson and Mathias 2000: 178). There is no analysis of why these problems may occur and how they might relate to the experiences of the individual.

'Body dysmorphic disorder' is also discussed in textbook B. The sufferer is described as believing that they have a body defect, when in reality, their physical appearance is normal. These preoccupations, according to the textbook, may become delusional, meaning that they will extend beyond a preoccupation with real or imaginary wrinkles and spots. The textbook describes how an individual with delusional ideas about their body will be diagnosed with a delusional disorder – *Somatic subtype*. There is no discussion of why this condition may occur and possibly relate to the individual's lived experience.

Textbook B discusses 'conversion disorder' and suggests that psychological desire or conflict is expressed through physiological means. It is considered that this process has two advantages for the individual. First, the person may avoid conscious awareness of a psychological conflict. Second, the person through exhibiting a bodily symptom such as paralysis will provide a legitimate reason for avoiding a situation or an event. The textbook suggests that individuals who present multiple somatic complaints without a medical explanation over several years may be diagnosed with 'somatisation disorder'. It acknowledges that a skilled practitioner may be able to pinpoint life or relationship problems as the foundation for such complaints. If complaints are mostly associated with the experience of pain, the patient may be diagnosed with 'somatoform pain disorder'.

Textbook A discusses the physical presentation of patients in terms of emphasising the importance of a well-maintained appearance. It states that socially, individuals have a responsibility to maintain a well-groomed appearance. Abandonment of such appearance is stated as frequent among patients suffering from mental illness. The distress experienced is regarded as being the cause of 'neglect' of personal grooming: 'This neglect is often inextricably linked to whatever mental illness the patient is suffering' (Brooking *et al.* 1992: 271). Suggestion as to means of reversing the neglect by patients of their body and clothing are formulated in terms of 'behavioural' psychological treatments. Under these programmes, self-grooming is rewarded with, for instance, edible items and privileges. Other programmes are also discussed. These encourage the patient to play an active part in monitoring, evaluating and correcting, 'deficiencies in their grooming and dress, and maintaining acceptable grooming behaviour' (ibid.). Bodily presentation is clearly considered in the textbook as relating closely to the psychiatric condition of the patient and as treatable as such.

Textbook B makes less emphasis upon the importance of acceptable appearance. It does however make links between a patient's appearance and their diagnosis. Patients who are diagnosed with schizophrenia for example, are described as inclined to neglect their self-care and are likely to collect and hoard rubbish or items, which have no relevance for the observer.

Bodily presentation is discussed in both textbooks with reference to eating disorders that are regarded as specific to women. The act of excessively controlling food intake in anorexia is described as having a desexualising effect on the sufferer who is considered to fear her sexuality. The psychological aspects of bulimia are also described. Depressive symptoms, low self-esteem and anger are considered as contributory factors. Sociocultural factors are considered, such as the cultural pressure upon young women to slim. Psychoanalytic theory is discussed in Textbook A, which is described as considering the fear of food as 'emphasising fears of oral impregnation' (ibid.: 414). Psychoanalytic theory is also discussed with emphasis upon the child–parent relation. The textbook states that many children lack self-esteem and self-worth as a result of their parents' failure to transmit these values. Biological causative factors are also discussed such as the 'hypothalamic dysfunction' theory.

## Summary of textbook findings

From examination of the above-cited nursing textbooks, it seems clear that awareness of sex differences is considered in their training and practice. Women's social position is considered to influence the onset of their mental illness, and the effects of socialisation leading to gender role stereotyping in relation to psychiatric diagnosis are also discussed. Feminine roles are considered to often have negative values attached to them, which frequently lead to women being diagnosed as mentally ill. In addition, the textbooks discuss sex differences in relation to psychiatric diagnosis. These sociological perspectives reveal the multidisciplinary focus of the pre-registration nursing course, and specifically the contribution of sociological thought which suggests a challenge to the psychiatric biomedical approach. There is emphasis upon women's social position and the experiences of women psychiatric patients but these are not given precedence over the medical model. With reference to eating difficulties, the textbooks acknowledge that these are predominantly a female phenomenon and, in addition, it considers that cultural values play a substantial part in influencing the ways in which women perceive their bodies. These considerations of the body as communicating conflicts stemming from cultural pressures challenge psychiatric medical methodology which formulates a predominantly biomedical basis to eating difficulties.

The textbook's discussion of eating disorders and dissociative disorder reveals a consideration of ways in which mental distress may be communicated through the body. It indicates that psychological factors may manifest themselves bodily as well as, or instead of, verbally. Furthermore, although nurses are taught about the importance of body language – their own body language rather than that of their patients – they are mostly taught about the body as cause not as language of mental illness.

## Conclusion

The textbooks used by psychiatrists and nurses in their training and practice place much emphasis upon the body. In their assessment of patients with mental illness, psychiatrists and nurses are encouraged to pay attention to physical appearance and presentation. Bodily presentation is also discussed in relation to the psychiatric conditions including 'depression', 'mania', 'eating disorders', 'schizophrenia' and 'dissociative disorder'. However, body presentations or symptoms are seen to merely relate to specific biologically determined mental illness, and are therefore considered within a biomedical framework. Another way to consider the physicality of people diagnosed with mental illness is to suggest that the body is a means by which patients seem to convey their life experience. As I stated in Chapter 1, words are often ineffective in the communication of distress especially for the person experiencing psychosis. In this context, the body seems to take on the role of communicator. The person is therefore saying something about their experience and as practitioners we tend to perceive these expressions as bizarre and *meaningless*. Consequently, the patient is never quite understood. I feel that the theoretical framework that most passionately articulates how symptoms often have meaning is psychoanalysis. Before I discuss this perspective, I shall first turn to feminist theories which, as we will see, do provide means for understanding the experiences of women, their bodies and mental illness.

# Chapter 4

# Women speaking

In the last chapter, following my discussion of Foucault's ideas, I outlined some brief examples of the focus upon the role of the body in the presentation of mental illness within British psychiatry. It has consistently focused upon bodily processes as cause of mental distress, on observation of the body, and on treatments in the form of therapies and procedures aimed at affecting the body. I examined contemporary texts used by psychiatrists and nurses in their training and clinical practice, and found that the texts used refer to a predominantly biomedical framework in their discussion of the understanding and treatment of mental illness and its bodily presentation.

There is currently a vast amount of literature on feminism and the body. In attempting to provide an understanding of women's mental distress, I have felt compelled to focus upon the 'second wave' feminist writings and subsequent writings on women and psychiatry, of the 1970s and 1980s. As I hope to demonstrate, these perspectives are relevant to many women's lives today. I know from my clinical experience that many women are still predominantly responsible for home-making, childcare and caring for dependent relatives. Consequently, women more frequently than men, experience social isolation and poverty, and these factors often contribute to their mental distress. Within the mental health system, there is often limited attention to women's life experiences in terms of their care of others.

I will now focus upon ways in which feminism has interpreted the body and in what ways its insights have been applied to understanding mental illness and its presentation. As I stated in the introduction, there is a vast range of writings on feminism and the body.[1] However, there is a very limited amount on the role of the female body and mental illness.[2] There are also a number of writings on women and mental illness, and although many discuss the ways in which historically, women's biology has been considered as responsible for their mental illness, they do not focus upon the body *specifically*. In my focus upon this issue, I have found that the work of the 'second wave' feminist writers of the 1970s and 1980s, and of subsequent writers on women and psychiatry, most appropriately address the experiences of women who encounter the mental health system today.

In this chapter, I will begin by discussing socialist/Marxist feminist accounts of women's oppression as a whole. Although they do not make explicit references to the body, they nevertheless describe the 'physical labour' of women in terms of their roles as mothers and carers, and its effects on women's sense of self. These ideas have been applied to women's mental distress by researchers such as Brown and Harris, and Ann Oakley. In this context, women's physical labour, stemming from outside cultural and economic pressures, has consequences for women's sense of self and their mental health. I will conclude this chapter by discussing radical feminism, which conceptualises women's oppression in terms of patriarchal control over women's bodies and sexuality. Subsequent writers, including Elaine Showalter, have applied these ideas to mental health practice. These writers reflect upon the outside violation of women's bodies by patriarchal structures and practices.

The ideas of the feminist writers I outline in this chapter were part of wider concerns relating to the position of women in the 1970s and early 1980s. However, it is clear that these concerns are still relevant today. A recent Department of Health strategy document, *Mainstreaming Gender and Women's Mental Health* (DH 2003), outlines how female mental health service users are asking for their mental distress to be understood in the context of their lives. Women are still predominantly responsible for home-making, childcare and caring for dependent relatives. In addition, more women than men experience sexual abuse, domestic violence and sexual violence (Williams *et al.* 1993; DH 2003). These factors appear to contribute to women's experiences of mental illness and within clinical practice there is often limited acknowledgement of these issues. These factors also seem to contribute to the distress of the two women patients I discuss in Chapter 8.[3] It is due to these factors that I have dedicated this chapter to women (and largely due to the fact that this book has as its foundation my PhD thesis in Women's Studies). The fact that mental health practice has consequences for male embodiment deserves much attention, but I do not cover this issue in this book. I do, however, briefly discuss male embodiment in relation to the case studies I present in Chapter 8.

The mental health practitioner may find it useful to think about the body and mental illness in relation to women in three ways. First, as I have stated, the 'physical labour' of women as carers for others and so forth, often contribute to their mental distress. This approach provides an alternative to the dominant biomedical explanations[4] of women's distress. Second, the ways in which psychiatric systems have sought to control the female body. Third, how women's distress is ultimately contained within, and expressed through, their bodies. The psychoanalytically minded French feminists, Luce Irigaray and Julia Kristeva, provide an understanding of this third point. However, I will deal with their work in Chapter 6 following my discussion of Freud and Lacan. I hope that the reader finds this chapter helpful in the understanding of the causes and context of women's mental illness at least from an economic, social and radical perspective and, if nothing else, learns something about the history of feminist thought along the way.

## Socialist/Marxist feminism

Although Marx made occasional references to women's social and economic situation, he did not create a coherent analysis of women's oppression. In *The Communist Manifesto*, Marx and Engels predicted that the abolition of the bourgeois family would end the way women are considered as mere child producers (Marx and Engels 1967: 101). However, Marx's concept of 'reproduction' was predominantly concerned with how social systems, particularly class structures, are reproduced throughout history.

Marxist feminists nevertheless argue that Marxism can be used to conceptualise women's oppression as being the result of social and economic structures within capitalist society. One central component of Marxist theory is that economic and social factors determine consciousness. This has been developed by Marxist feminists in the understanding of women's social subordination to men. They draw upon this concept to explain the way in which women, in their multifaceted roles, create a concept of themselves that would otherwise fail to exist if they did not encounter social and economic subordination both at home and in the workplace (Holmstrom 1984: 464).

The Marxist economic perspective identifies the unequal power dynamics behind the transactions between the bourgeoisie and proletariat within capitalist society. An exploitative system is identified whereby the bourgeoisie employers control the means of production, and the proletariat must choose between their own exploitation or being without work. Marxist feminists incorporate a gender aspect to this analysis. Restricted in their child rearing responsibilities, women are often victims of low wages and are more likely to be exploited by their male colleagues.

Another key Marxist term is that of 'alienation', which describes how class distinction and human separation at work, such as on an assembly line, lead to loss of a unity of human experience. Applying this concept to women, Ann Foreman describes how men are able to seek relief from their experiences of alienation within their relations with women at home. Women's experiences of alienation however, according to Foreman, are more profound. The basic foundations of their oppression exist within their intimate relations with men. Foreman states that women have a social and psychological persona within capitalism based around the fulfilment of the needs of others, and if this were to cease it would leave women without a sense of self (1977: 101).

Socialist feminists such as Juliet Mitchell, Sheila Rowbotham and Michelle Barrett have made a number of criticisms of classical Marxist theory, focusing on what Heidi Hartmann refers to as its 'sex-blind' (Hartmann in Tong 1989: 180) tendencies, and its inadequacy in addressing economic, social and cultural factors specific to women. Socialist feminism considers the importance of gender as well as of class in the analysis of women's oppression. Rosemarie Tong states that socialist feminism can be considered as 'the confluence of Marxist, radical and, more arguably, psychoanalytic streams of feminist thought' (1989: 173).

In texts such as *Women's Estate* (1971), Mitchell criticises Marxist feminist analysis for solely linking women's oppression to their relationship to economic production. She emphasises that women's reproductive function has escaped the attention of Marxist analysis. Mitchell argues that reproduction, the socialisation of children and female sexuality are of equal importance to a consideration of women's relationship to economic production, in the understanding of women's oppression. She emphasises the necessity for change in all four structures in order to eliminate female oppression: 'Economic demands are still primary, but must be accompanied by coherent policies for the other three elements (reproduction, sexuality and socialization)' (1971: 100). Mitchell disagrees with the Marxist notion that the elimination of patriarchy and the family as an economic unit would follow the overthrow of capitalism. According to Mitchell, patriarchy is reinforced through culture and the unconscious, therefore a psychic as well as a material revolution is necessary for the liberation of women.

In *Women's Consciousness, Man's World* (1973) Rowbotham argues that Marxist theory fails to acknowledge women's personal experience of oppression, and suggests that women experience oppression through the process of language and culture, as well as through economic factors. As a class group, women encounter damaging psychological consequences of their subordination. Considered as 'carers', women are given a 'peculiar kind of respect as long as they fulfil their role' (1973: 77). Rowbotham states that women's roles are multiple and often oppressive, and frequently women feel isolated. Care and sentiment are not considered as appropriate in the social world and are out of context within the male workplace. Therefore, women bear the weight of this sentiment and a distortion takes place within the family. This can lead to love being seen as a possession, and tenderness as submission, which can cause violence. Women, according to Rowbotham, in their multiple caring roles, effectively provide capitalism with the 'human relations it cannot maintain in the world of men's work' (ibid.).

Rowbotham acknowledges that one of the numerous roles women undertake within the family is that of housewife. She applies the Marxist term 'false consciousness' to housework. She argues that housework has no labour contract, and women internalise the idea that domestic, wifely tasks are carried out because of love. According to Rowbotham, housework has been largely ignored by Marxist theory with its emphasis upon surplus value within the capitalist mode of production. Rowbotham states that women are placed within the family mode of production that is controlled differently. She states that housework does not constitute what is considered as real work, and escapes the attention of economic calculation.

Michelle Barrett highlights the family as a site of women's oppression, and the tendency of Marxist theory to ignore this. She states how, historically, popular ideology has considered the family as 'essentially and naturally there' (1980: 187), thus reinforcing social constructions of gender identity in which women are considered as 'naturally' nurturing and caring. Consequently, the family or the 'family-household system' restricts women's access to paid labour by reinforcing ideologies about their role as reproducers, and their servile position to men. This leads to the sexual division of labour as women's roles in the workplace and in the home are considered to reflect each other.

## Brown and Harris: the Camberwell study

Marxist and socialist feminist thought has identified economic, social and cultural factors behind women's oppression. Specifically it has focused on women's role in the domestic sphere and generational reproduction. Those investigating the contributing factors to women's mental distress have also considered such factors. Brown and Harris, for example, conducted an intensive study of clinically depressed women in the area of Camberwell in the late 1970s. They consider that preceding research, which had attempted to link social factors to the onset of psychiatric conditions, was inadequate. According to Brown and Harris, such studies failed to link 'in a persuasive and testable way' (1978: 17), factors such as social class, sex and sex roles, and specific life events such as loss of an intimate relationship, with depressive conditions. As an alternative, Brown and Harris focused upon a specific research model of inquiry made up of three components.

The first component of the Brown and Harris research model refers to specific 'provoking agents' relating to the onset of depression. These include life events such as bereavement, loss of employment, and ongoing 'difficulties' such as having to deal with family members experiencing alcoholism and unemployment. Brown and Harris state that although these are obviously distressing events, they do not in themselves greatly influence the onset of depression and fail to address the marked differences between different social groups in rates of depression. Consequently, Brown and Harris introduce the second component of their research model, namely, what they called 'vulnerability factors'.

Brown and Harris suggest that in addition to experiencing a 'provoking agent', certain individuals also experience 'vulnerability factors' that increase their susceptibility to depression. For example, lack of employment can further increase the risk of developing depression once a major loss has occurred, such as loss of a husband. During the course of their research, Brown and Harris found that the following 'vulnerability factors' increased women's probability of developing depression: 'Loss of mother before eleven', 'presence at home of three or more children under fourteen', 'absence of a confiding relationship', and 'a lack of a full or part-time job' (ibid.: 179).

The third research model component is 'symptom formation'. According to Brown and Harris, these factors do not increase the possibility of developing depression, but nevertheless influence the severity of the depression. For example, Brown and Harris found that loss of a mother before the age of eleven may increase the possibility of developing depression. However, the actual experience and circumstances of the event influence the severity of the depression. For example, Brown and Harris state that the mother may be lost by death, or by other circumstances such as adoption, which may have less emotional impact.

Brown and Harris found that social class played a significant role in explaining differences in the rates of depression. They report upon the chronic difficulties faced by working-class women who were found to be more likely to experience one or more of the three established 'vulnerability factors'. In addition, the women were more likely to experience severe life events and long-term major difficulties, particularly if they had children at home, housing problems, financial difficulties and relationship problems with a husband or children.

The findings of this study are substantial in highlighting links between social factors such as class, housing and employment, and rates of depression in women. The researchers suggest their study provides the need for concern with the position of women within the family system and 'the role of women in the wider economy and the values given to these functions by the media and society at large' (ibid.: 291).

## The plight of the housewife

Joan Busfield in *Men, Women and Madness* (1996) states that the image of the trapped housewife suggested by three of Brown and Harris's vulnerability factors initiated many feminist writers such as Ann Oakley and Betty Friedan to consider the factors influencing mental distress in women (Busfield 1996: 200). Oakley's research in 1974 on the experiences of housewives was successful in revealing the repetitive, monotonous and lonely nature of the role. Oakley began her book, *Housewife* (1974) by describing the status of housewives within industrialised society. First, the role is considered as exclusively female. Second, it is associated with women being economically dependent upon their husbands within the marital relationship. Third, the work undertaken is considered as non-work, whereby the woman receives no salary and is not entitled to financial benefits such as sickness or unemployment benefit. Fourth, the role of house-wife takes precedence over the other roles in a woman's life. Oakley states that women's ties to domestic responsibilities curtail any progression toward equality between the sexes.

Oakley's research aimed to highlight the dissatisfaction of women's ties to the 'private' sphere of the home, by interviewing housewives and providing four case studies. She found that the role of housewife brought about isolation and loss of personal identity for women. Women's dissat-isfaction with their domestic roles was often expressed verbally. Of her social isolation, one woman stated: 'Not knowing anybody else you tend to get this feeling that unless you go out and talk to someone, you'll go stark raving mad' (Oakley 1974: 101). Oakley found, however, that many housewives also expressed their feelings indirectly, through anxiety symptoms such as nervousness, insomnia, and drug- and alcohol-related difficulties. It seems, then, that the women interviewed by Oakley expressed their distress through bodily means. Oakley reports that such symptoms are recognised as the 'housewife's disease' (ibid.: 232) by *The International Yearbook of Neurology, Psychiatry and Neurosurgery* in 1974. She states that symptoms such as agoraphobia, nervous breakdowns, heart palpitations and fainting were found by a US study to be more common in full-time housewives as opposed to employed women and men. The study also revealed that between 1957 and 1967 an increase in consumption of psychotropic drugs, such as sedatives and anti-depressants, occurred. Three-quarters of the consumers were found to be women.

Oakley suggests that women's traditional roles within the domestic sphere have led to their dissatisfaction and isolation. This dissatisfaction is often expressed covertly, and may take the form of depression and anxiety states in women. Oakley suggests that this 'circle of learnt depri-vation' is centred upon family life within which women are given no other status than that associated with domesticity. She proposed that political action on the part of women, which challenges both personal relationships and bureaucratic structures, was required in order for change to occur.

## Family troubles and mental health

The 1988 research conducted by Agnes Miles consists of a study based on 200 interviews with sixty-five women and twenty men between the ages of twenty and fifty-five. Miles states that the focus of the study is one that compares the experiences of the women participants with that of the men. The greater number of women participants in the study reflects epistemo-logical findings which conclude that women are more frequently diagnosed as 'neurotic' than men. The participants were all suffering from conditions such as 'depression', 'phobia', 'obsessive-compulsive disorders' and 'anxiety states'. These conditions are collectively defined under the psychiatric category of 'neurosis'. Following their diagnosis, the participants all received psychiatric treatment on an outpatient basis consisting of regular contact with a psychiatrist, prescribed medication and other contacts such as day centres. The first interviews focused on the ways in which participants made sense of their neurosis, and the factors that were perceived as influential to its onset.

Half of the women interviewed spoke of experiences of an unhappy marriage as influential on the onset of their symptoms. Although many of these women described experiences of violent, unsupportive and inconsiderate behaviour from their husbands, many nevertheless stated that they, too, were responsible for such situations. One woman for example, said: 'I know I should shout back and stand up for myself, but I can't . . . it's not my fault, but it's not his either, really, he can't help being what he is' ('Bridget' in Miles 1988: 29). Miles concludes that this is typical of many women's responses to a violent or aggressive partner. She states that studies that examine women's experiences of sexual violence frequently reveal the ways in which they see themselves as partly to blame for their partner's behaviour, or as provoking the attack made against them.

Strained and difficult family relationships were also perceived as contributing to the onset of neurotic symptoms. Another major factor, reported by thirteen women, was the caring for sick or disabled relatives for a period of several years. One woman reported how having to care for her two mentally handicapped children left her feeling guilt at letting her other two children down. Another woman stated how she looked after her terminally ill father until his death. In the eighteen months in which she cared for him she never left the house. Her only other contacts were brief visits from the neighbour who did the shopping, and the doctor. Following her father's death, this process continued: 'I panicked at the thought of leaving the house. It was only then I knew it was agoraphobia' ('Kate' in Miles 1988: 34).

It is invariably women who take sole responsibility for the nursing and care of sick family members, as Miles states:

> Much evidence has been accumulated about the nursing role of women. Sick children are nursed by their mothers, disabled and mentally ill relatives are looked after by the women of the family, and geriatric parents are nursed by daughters and daughters-in-law.
>
> (Miles 1988: 34)

Miles reports how research has pinpointed the psychological harm done to women who perform caring roles, specifically those who care for a mentally ill relative. Such women are perceived to neglect their own health because of the numerous responsibilities they are required to take on in the care of others.

In a similar vein to Oakley's interviews of housewives during the 1970s, Miles states how the women in her study spoke of the isolation and stress associated with the undertaking of housework. The women reported long hours, isolation from a wider social network, and sole responsibility for family health which often led to obsessive cleaning as one woman reported how she cleaned the sink six or seven times a day, and still thought it was dirty. Some women, although burdened with such domestic roles, felt a pressure to stay at home due to family demands, and the low self-esteem they experienced as a result of being tied to the home for long periods. Additionally, receiving the label 'neurotic' added further pressures to stay at home as any potential self-esteem was consequently banished.

The women participants also focused on specific life events such as bereavement as explanations for their neuroses. Physical conditions such as PMT and the menopause, were occasionally cited as contributory factors, but more specifically the women frequently reported that they had experienced difficulty in convincing men such as their husbands, and doctors, of the physical and psychological discomfort they often experienced. Other factors identified stemmed from childhood experiences as one woman reported her jealousy of her brother, which led to her breakdown while she was preparing for 'A' levels. However, Miles found overall that these factors were given less emphasis by the women, in comparison to those experienced within the domestic sphere consisting of the care of the home, children and relatives.

The men of the Miles study, by contrast, did not tend to consider their marital relationships, or family relationships as contributing to the onset of their neurosis. Their focus was directed away from the domestic sphere towards two factors: work-related problems and physical illness. One man, for example, reported how he was off sick for a year and consequently lost his job and the company he worked for placed him in another position with less money and status, which he perceived as contributing to his distress. Other men considered that physical factors such as undergoing operations, or heart or chest problems influenced the onset of their symptoms.

The men and women of the Miles study were interviewed a year after their initial diagnosis. They were each asked to discuss any changes or improvements taking place, and any existing difficulties. Miles devises four categories in order to assess their current situation: 'quite recovered', 'improved', 'unchanged' and 'worse than a year previously'. Of the women participants, who were the first group to be assessed, fourteen perceived themselves as being 'quite recovered' meaning that they were clear of neurotic symptoms, nineteen were 'improved' which meant experiencing occasional symptoms, twenty women were 'unchanged', and twelve stated that they were 'worse than a year previously'.

The women who reported complete or partial recovery had each experienced a major change in their lives such as moving home, gaining employment, being relieved of being responsible for the care of a sick or disabled family member, and divorce or separation. Nine of the women, for example, were divorced or separated which brought consequences such as becoming the main provider by gaining employment, or claiming welfare benefit. Other women moved house to areas with better supportive social networks and amenities. Some had been enduring dire housing conditions such as dampness, so a move in itself was perceived by them to be beneficial for their mental health. Gaining employment or moving from domestic work at home into paid employment brought about, according to Miles, 'greater job satisfaction, the companionship of congenial adults and the confidence that comes from earning money' (ibid.: 146).

The women who reported that their neurotic symptoms were unchanged or worse, clearly lacked, according to Miles, the life changes and supportive networks that appeared to so blatantly aid the previous group: 'among the women who reported no improvement, beneficial life-events were almost entirely absent' (ibid.: 153). Some of the women reporting no improvement had either terminated their psychiatric treatment themselves, or had been discharged. This invariably meant that they returned to their GP and were prescribed further medication for their continuing symptoms. Miles reports that many of these women appeared resigned to their circumstances and were further discouraged from making changes due to apparent rejection from supportive networks.

Of the twenty men interviewed, five stated recovery, nine improvement, three no change and three worsened symptoms. They perceived improvements in terms of employment; many had resumed their old jobs after a period of sick leave, or had obtained new jobs. The men did not experience the life changes the women associated with recovery. None were divorced, for instance, and only one moved house. Miles concludes that the men's reports of greater improvement as compared to that of the women may have been due to their difficulty in expressing vulnerability. However, improvements were more likely to be due to better marital support and a greater effort on the part of the psychiatrist and those involved in their care.

Miles' study gives evidence for the suggestion that, as she puts it, 'neurosis is a social disorder lending itself to social remedies' (ibid.: 154). It certainly appears clear from this work that social remedies are obviously of benefit to women in their frequent confinement to the domestic sphere. However, there are a number of points that require further investigation. Many of the women who Miles interviewed clearly stated how they felt solely or partly responsible for their experiences of unhappy relationships, consisting of aggressive acts and sexual violence. It would be interesting to examine the processes behind this. Similarly, in situations whereby a relative is sick and requires care, the women seemed to accept and not question sole responsibility. Perhaps this requires examination of the wider structures of society that serve to place, and justify the position of, women in such roles.

A psychoanalytic understanding may also be useful to understand why women readily see themselves as responsible for the behaviour and care of others, and how this is perhaps unconsciously reproduced. The work of Nancy Chodorow for example, examines how women 'become' mothers, which is influenced by the sexual division of labour within culture and its effects on the psychological development of children. Chodorow states, 'In a society where mothers provide nearly exclusive care and certainly the most meaningful relationship to the infant, the infant develops its sense of self mainly in relation to her' (1978: 78). Chodorow argues that girls internalise caring roles from their identification with their mothers. She focuses upon the pre-Oedipal phase of development where the mother is the central focus. Girls, according to Chorodow, develop a sense of self that is continuous with others, and is the foundation of their need to mother and care for others. In contrast, boys reject the mothering, nurturing aspects of themselves in order to identify with their fathers. In the Miles study, emphasis upon the early development of the participants was rather overshadowed by the emphasis upon social factors. Perhaps it is important to consider the importance of early experiences and their effects on the individual's psyche, which subsequent social and economic difficulties may exacerbate.

## Psychological burdens and domestic labour

Although full-time housewives are decreasing in number, Lesley Doyal points out that the psychological burdens such as low status, associated with domestic labour, 'continue to be important issues in explaining women's mental health problems' (1995: 37). In a similar vein to the work of Brown and Harris, and of Oakley and Miles, Doyal's book, *What Makes Women Sick?* published in 1995, cites the high prevalence of depression in housewives, especially those with young children. She goes on to state how mothering itself, according to several studies, can be accompanied by depression and anxiety despite society's message that it is greatly enjoyable and rewarding. Doyal suggests that mental health problems can result from women losing their individual identity upon becoming mothers.

Research carried out in the UK and US reveal, according to Doyal, a consistent presentation of ways in which women's ties to domestic labour and family responsibilities often make them susceptible to developing mental health problems. Doyal states that, in order to assess the extent of this problem, it is necessary to examine ethnographic research carried out in different social contexts. She outlines research published in 1987[5] by Helen Ulrich who compared the experiences of depression between affluent, married women in South India, and women in the UK and US, such as those discussed in the Brown and Harris study.

Several women in the south Indian village studied by Ulrich reported loss of a parent at an early age, as did the women of the Brown and Harris study. However, this loss in the Indian sample was found to be as a result of marriage customs rather than death, and the women's powerlessness in deciding their own destinies. Daughters moving to another village as a result of arranged marriages often reported distress at losing previous close ties with family and friends, which were difficult to resume in new surroundings, whereby they were confined to the domestic sphere. The mothers who were left behind when their daughters moved away also reported loss and isolation.

Ulrich found, however, that the most frequently reported cause of depression was widowhood. The death of a husband is, according to Ulrich, a loss most feared. The personal support of a husband was perceived by the women as a great loss, but more specifically there were losses of identity and status. These women had practically no status without their husbands. Their identity had been intrinsically tied up with their husband's existence.

Many of the younger women of the next generation in the village had encountered greater freedoms. These involved better educational opportunities, a greater say in the everyday running of their lives and increased opportunities for working outside of the home. This, according to Ulrich, resulted in lower rates of depression among the younger women.

This research reveals how women's experiences of mental distress cross cultural boundaries. Universally, they are perceived as responsible for the daily care of the home, children and relatives, which, in turn, makes them susceptible to depression. In a similar vein to Miles' research, Ulrich concludes by stating that when women are relieved of their ties to the domestic sphere, and are offered greater social opportunities, such as better social networks, education and paid employment outside the home, they suffer less mental distress.

## Mental illness and the wider social order

Joan Busfield emphasises the importance of social factors in explaining the prevalence of mental distress in women. However, she stresses that it is also necessary to explore the meanings attached to concepts of mental illness in relation to gender, and the social structures in which men and women exist:

> Although the evidence of the impact of social factors in generating mental disorder (as currently constituted) is very strong, a focus on the specific structural features of men's and women's lives, and the meanings attached to them, is more fruitful.
>
> (Busfield 1996: 8)

Busfield therefore draws upon the work of Foucault in examining how 'discourses' of mental illness are constructed and reinforced and serve to produce knowledge. Busfield applies a gender analysis to Foucault's concepts.

According to Busfield, concepts of mental illness are intrinsically part of the wider social order that serves to give meaning to differing aspects of social behaviour. Drawing upon the work of Foucault, Busfield states that varying mental illnesses 'are concepts that set the boundaries of un-reason' (ibid.: 232) that threaten to disrupt the social order. According to Busfield, the concept of unreason is essentially gendered, as women are culturally associated with it. Women are perceived as passive, irrational and emotional, and therefore as not responsible for their actions, whereas men are seen as staying within the boundaries of reason and rationality, and their behaviour is considered to be something for which they are responsible. This has negative consequences for both sexes. Women's apparent powerlessness, irrationality and emotionality, concepts kept in place by social institutions, serve to justify male power. Consequently, women are more easily and more frequently diagnosed and treated as mentally ill. Busfield states:

> Women's relative lack of power in many situations in comparison with men, and the perceptions surrounding their lack of power, means they are doubly disadvantaged . . . their lack of power makes it more likely that their behaviours may be viewed as indicative of mental disorder.
>
> (1996: 236)

It is therefore necessary to focus upon ways in which wider social factors influence the prevalence of mental illness in women. A commitment to decreasing unemployment, and the provision of better education and child-care services are necessary. In addition, as Busfield suggests, attention that moves from focusing on just the individual with mental illness, to one that focuses upon the wider social institutions of psychiatry is also necessary. Better regulation in order to prevent the abuse and exploitation of patients, of which a high proportion are women is required. However, as well as these important proposals, Busfield states that any analysis of the relation between gender and mental illness, requires an examination of the ways in which the very discourses of mental illness are perceived and judged, and how women fit into this framework.

The research I have outlined above raises some important points for the understanding of the prevalence of mental distress in women. These perspectives focus upon the importance of understanding mental distress and its presentation in a wider social context beyond a purely biomedical emphasis. Women's ties to the domestic sphere and often sole responsibility for the care of children and relatives undoubtedly contribute to making them susceptible to mental distress, especially if there is additional social and economic hardship such as poverty and unemployment. It is striking that the conclusions reached by Brown and Harris, and others in the 1970s, still appear to have relevance. As I said above, I will demonstrate in my observations of, and interactions with, women mental health patients in Chapter 8, that their ties to the domestic sphere and their hard physical work can be seen as contributing to their experiences of mental distress.

## Radical feminism

I will now turn to radical feminist perspectives on women's position in society, which can be divided into two areas. Those exemplified by Kate Millett and Andrea Dworkin consider gender roles and the patriarchal control of women's bodies and sexuality. The second area, exemplified by Shulamith Firestone and Adrienne Rich, considers reproduction and mothering.

Kate Millett in her book, *Sexual Politics*, published in 1970, proposes that women's oppression has its foundations in a patriarchal system that places men into masculine roles such as those espousing domination and strength, and women into feminine roles of passivity and emotionality that serve to keep them subordinate to men. Millett states that these separate roles are reinforced by beliefs about men and women's 'natural' characteristics that stem from their biological make up: Millett states: 'culture consents to believe the possession of the male indicator, the testes, penis, and scrotum, in itself characterises the aggressive impulse ... the same process of reinforcement is evident in producing the chief "feminine" virtue of passivity' (1970: 31). She suggests that all power relations are based on this male–female model of male control. For the liberation of women, male control and the placing of men and women into distinct gender roles in order to subordinate and oppress them need to be eliminated.

Millett emphasises that the roles of masculinity and femininity are social constructs. Accordingly, what is seen in society to constitute masculinity and femininity is learnt and internalised through socialisation. The notions associated with such gender differentiation operate and are reinforced in all economic and social structures, such as the family.

This process has implications for how both men and women perceive themselves. Children are encouraged to think and behave in certain ways in order to comply with the gender expectations placed upon them. We shall see how this process is apparent in the patients I observe and interview in Chapter 8. The women, in particular, appear to suggest that they do not live up to the roles expected of them, for instance as wives and mothers. Millett suggests that for women to survive within the patriarchal system, it is best for them to display actions and behaviour considered to be feminine, or alternatively if they reject the feminine role they will encounter cruelty, rejection and intimidation from men.

Women's confinement to the feminine role, secured and justified both culturally and socially, is responsible for their oppression. For changes to occur, women must free themselves from this role. Millett proposes an androgynous future whereby men and women would exist in separate subcultures. She states that the separate values once associated with masculinity and femininity should be challenged. All characteristics once associated with both genders could be incorporated within the androgynous psyche and given equal value.

Andrea Dworkin in her book, *Pornography: Men Possessing Women* (1979), proposes that pornography can be seen as an example of male control of the female body and sexuality. She proposes that male power, which permeates all aspects of culture, is the root of female oppression whereby men exert their greater physical strength to gain power over women. According to Dworkin, men have a sense of self, which is reinforced and confirmed by society, in terms of its male-centred practices and structures. The male sense of self also enables men to feel entitled to take whatever they want freely. Women, by contrast, lack a sense of self and have never been able to define their own identity and needs. Men possess the power to name and define feminine behaviour. If women reject the feminine role, it leads to dire consequences for them, and this is evident in male-controlled structures including psychiatry, and in the case of male violence against women.

With reference to male sexual power, Dworkin somewhat depressingly defines it as the control of female sexuality that is reinforced within culture: 'Male sexual power is the substance of culture. It resonates everywhere. The celebration of rape in story, song, and science is a paradigmatic articulation of male sexual power as a cultural absolute' (ibid.: 23). She states that the male control of female sexuality is prevalent in the sexually explicit and degrading portrayals of women in pornography. Other aspects of male power are also highlighted in pornography such as male control over its production and distribution. Dworkin states that women in society are valued in the same way as the women portrayed within pornography, and its existence signifies oppression.

It is harrowing reading the work of Dworkin. In writing about pornography, she would often include many examples of pornographic literature. It is easy to find these rather exciting and titillating. But one is constantly reminded by Dworkin that they are gruesomely oppressive and violent against the female sex. I wonder if this is one of the problems with pornographic *literature*. We perhaps intrinsically know it belittles women. But if we enjoy it, does this mean we unavoidably support the objectification of women and their bodies?

## Women's biology as restriction

Shulamith Firestone in *The Dialectic of Sex*, suggests that women's oppression has its foundations in the biological differences between the sexes: 'It was woman's reproductive biology that accounted for her original and continued oppression' (1970: 74). Firestone proposes that women's reproductive capabilities have been the cause of their oppression throughout history, leading her to revise Marx and Engels' concept of historical materialism from a feminist perspective. For Marx and Engels, it is the class struggle between the bourgeoisie and proletariat that constitutes movement in history. Firestone, however, proposes that it is rather the struggle between males and females, and a biological analysis of women's subordination is therefore necessary, rather than one that solely considers their economic position as emphasised by Marxist and socialist feminists.

Even if women encounter better legal, educational and economic freedoms, Firestone proposes, unless they are freed from their reproductive roles, they will never experience liberation. The restrictive opposites of masculinity and femininity, and women's restrictive ties to the domestic sphere as mothers and homemakers, will never be abandoned unless patriarchal reproduction as well as capitalist production is abolished. Consequently, a biological revolution, whereby women's reproductive functions would be replaced by technology, is the solution. With sophisticated artificial means of reproduction, women would be freed from feminine roles that enslave them. Firestone states that this would have consequences for capitalism. She highlights that the biological family has served to keep capitalism intact, and the fact that women reproduce enables capitalism to confine women to the private domestic sphere.

However, with technology replacing reproduction, the family would not survive as an economic unit. Technology can also serve to aid the means of production, which would result in men and women no longer having to endure separate reproductive and productive roles. The abandonment of distinct productive and reproductive roles for men and women would mean that all oppressive power relations would be overcome, such as between capitalist and worker, and master and slave. The first sperm banks opened in Iowa City and Tokyo in 1964, and they were opening commercially at the time Firestone was writing in the 1970s in the US. Were these perhaps the first steps towards a reduction in distinct reproductive roles for men and women?

In Firestone's estimation, patriarchy has been responsible for the myth of pregnancy and motherhood as idyllic experiences. She refers to pregnancy at its best as barely tolerable, and at its worst as a barbaric experience. Furthermore, she proposes that the very function of motherhood is responsible for the generation of jealousy and possessiveness within human relations. In order to create a society where divisions and hierarchies are abolished, the act of favouring one's own offspring over another due to its evolution from one's own ovum or sperm must be overcome.

Adrienne Rich, in *Of Woman Born* (1976), disagrees with Firestone's complete disavowal of motherhood and states that women could celebrate their reproductive capabilities and experiences, if they were able to reclaim mothering from patriarchal culture. Rich suggests that men are profoundly jealous of women's reproductive capabilities and ability to give life. Men are rather fearful that the ability to give life is coupled with an ability to bring death. Thus, they see women's reproductive functions as strange and fearful and something requiring control.

As a consequence of this fear, Rich suggests, men have controlled women's reproduction. For example, male obstetricians and obstetrical forceps took over from women midwives and their less technological practices. Male doctors produce rules and literature on how women should look, feel and act during pregnancy and childbirth: 'Women have been both mothers and daughters, but have written little on the subject, the vast majority of literary and visual images of motherhood comes to us filtered through a collective or individual male consciousness' (Rich 1976: 61). According to Rich, these rules often counteract women's real experiences that subsequently make pregnancy alienating to them. If women were able to fully reclaim their actual experiences and take back the control from men, they may encounter the powers associated with their reproductive capabilities.

While Marxist and socialist feminisms perceive women's oppression as stemming from economic and social structures associated with capitalism, radical feminism emphasises an oppressive patriarchal system that imposes gender roles and controls female sexuality and mothering roles. Many of the issues raised by radical feminist thought regarding patriarchy (as opposed to capital and class) have been applied to women and mental distress, notably by Phyllis Chesler in her book, *Women and Madness*.

## The paradoxical position of women

Chesler's 1972 study of women in American psychiatric institutions examined sex role stereotyping whereby women are considered as possessing characteristics such as emotionality, dependency and passivity. According to Chesler, these feminine characteristics are considered negatively within culture, which results in women being diagnosed as mad.[6] Furthermore, if women reject these female roles this, too, is perceived as mad. Chesler states that women are, therefore, subject to the paradoxical position whereby they are considered mad if they comply with the devalued female role and also considered mad if they reject this role.

The starting point in Chesler's analysis is to highlight ways in which male and female behaviour is defined and given meaning. Men, she states, are less likely to be labelled as mad than women, even if they exhibit disturbed behaviour:

> Many men *are* severely 'disturbed' – but the form their 'disturbance' takes is either not seen as 'neurotic' or is not treated by psychiatric incarceration. Theoretically, all men, but especially white, wealthy, and older men, can act out many 'disturbed' (and non-'disturbed') drives more easily than women can.
>
> (1997: 78)

Women however, are treated with less tolerance. Societal conditioning expects women in their female roles to exhibit emotional distress, but this is not received with understanding and empathy. According to Chesler, such behaviour is perceived as childlike and something to be managed rather than praised. Furthermore, such behaviour is managed with psychiatric procedures such as ECT, excessive medication and prolonged incarceration in psychiatric hospitals.

Theorists, including Goffman and Foucault, emphasise the patriarchal aspects of psychiatric institutions, and have observed that what goes on inside these institutions reflects the wider structures of patriarchal oppression. With reference to these observations, Chesler states that women's experiences within psychiatric confinement often reflect their experiences within the family. She states that women are often poorly nurtured as children and are then refused mothering by men as adults. As a consequence, women often crave the 'mothering' aspects of hospitalisation and embark upon 'psychiatric careers' more readily than men. Women often, Chesler proposes, feel rather at home within hospitals and frequently think that they will receive love from the nurses and attendants caring for them. However, according to Chesler, these 'mothers' do not 'like' women patients. Furthermore, institutional mothers cannot, as in the case of real mothers, protect their daughters from the violence and rape Chesler reports as frequently occurring within psychiatric institutions.

The mothering aspects of institutionalisation involve women patients being punished if they reject the feminine role. Chesler suggests that women who are more cautious or ambivalent about rejecting their feminine roles often wish to be punished in order to be saved from the dire consequences that may follow. Psychiatric institutions can be seen to take on the role of punishing women into submission and compliance. If women succeed in rejecting their sex roles by becoming angry and aggressive they are further punished with medication and psychiatric methods and practices.

According to Chesler, most clinicians who write about, treat and diagnose women psychiatric patients are responsible for reinforcing the devalued female role. She outlines a 1970 study by I.K. Broverman *et al.*, which investigates the attitudes of a group of mental health practitioners.

The group was asked to examine the behaviours that characterise a mentally healthy man, a mentally healthy woman or a mentally healthy adult independent of sex. The finding of the study reported that the characteristics of a healthy adult matched that of a man, but not that of a woman. Chesler concludes that this reveals how women are perceived as mentally unhealthy if they stay within the female role, and likewise if they step out of it.

I will now continue to examine how the ideas about patriarchy have been applied to women's mental distress through looking at the work of Elaine Showalter and Diane Hudson.

## Prevailing ideas of femininity and psychiatric practice

Elaine Showalter's fascinating 1985 book, *The Female Malady* provides a history of psychiatry from a feminist perspective. She identifies how madness has been perceived as a predominantly female condition. Furthermore, the cultural images of desirable and appropriate feminine behaviour have been synonymous, she says, with popular perceptions of madness. Such images do not merely reflect prevailing scientific and medical ideas, but contribute to the cultural framework in which ideas about femininity and insanity were constructed.

She argues that at the end of the eighteenth century perceptions regarding the care of the mad, and perceptions of madness, changed. The mad had previously been seen in male terms as brutish and grotesque. The introduction of asylums by English social reformers replaced harsher treatments in prisons, workhouses and privately run madhouses. It was considered that moral guidance and benevolence were more appropriate treatments and this marked the introduction of asylums and humanitarian approaches. This transition changed perceptions of madness from being predominantly male to female. As the nineteenth century unfolded, 'the appealing madwoman gradually displaced the repulsive madman, both as prototype of the confined lunatic and as a cultural icon' (Showalter 1985: 8).

The conception of madness as a female phenomenon was reflected in a range of cultural images of the early nineteenth century. Showalter shows how female irrationality, for example, which was perceived as endearing, appears in works such as George Dyer's sonnet *Written in Bedlam: On Seeing a Beautiful Young Female Maniac* (1801). The Romantic artists and writers portray the most culturally prevalent images of mad women. Mad women feature, for instance, as Walter Scott's heroine Lucy, Shakespeare's Ophelia, and Crazy Jane originally portrayed by Matthew Lewis in 1793. The character of Lucy portrays female sexuality as dangerous, untameable and a violent force against men. Ophelia represents the perceived femininity of madness. Showalter states: 'Even her death by drowning has associations with the feminine and the irrational, since water is the organic symbol of woman's fluidity: blood, milk, tears' (Showalter 1985: 11). Crazy Jane is represented as being abandoned by her lover and consequently retreating into madness. Showalter argues that she stands for female vulnerability and the perceived female reliance upon the affection of a man.

These cultural images had a profound effect upon social perceptions of the relationship between femininity and madness, which, in turn, influenced how women were treated within the psychiatric asylums of the time. Showalter identifies deliberate attempts to keep women in the feminine role, and to also curb the desires and wayward expressions of women. An obvious indication of the perceived connections between madness and the feminine was to be identified in the numbers of women patients now exceeding the numbers of men. By 1872, 'out of 58,640 certified lunatics in England and Wales, 31,822 were women' (ibid.: 52). The fact that more women than men were admitted into asylums provoked much debate among Victorian psychiatrists. Although factors such as poverty and child rearing were considered as causative factors, the dominant viewpoint was one that identified an innate female instability connected to female reproductive capacities. Menarche was considered to bring the first threat of insanity, and control of menstruation was deemed necessary for good mental health. The attempt to control the reproductive cycle suggests to Showalter, a fear of female sexuality on the part of male psychiatrists.

The perceived obscenity of female patients served to shock the asylum doctors and male patients, and was considered to require harsh treatment. The prevailing thought was that if women's bodies in terms of their reproductive cycles were controlled, this, in turn, would manage their minds. Clitoridectomy, devised by Dr Issac Baker Brown of the London Obstetrical Society, was a regular treatment for female insanity. Brown suggested that madness in women was caused by masturbation. By the 1860s Brown extended his surgical techniques to the removal of the labia. Brown made a point of performing surgery on women expressing a wish to make use of the newly introduced Divorce Act of 1857. Many of his patients, who were considered insane because of disobedient or impulsive behaviour, became reclusive and submissive following the operation. Several of them proceeded to passively devote their lives to marriage and child rearing. Brown's other patients often complained that they were often manipulated into having the treatment. Consequently, these complaints led to him being expelled from the Obstetrical Society for the misuse of male authority.

Physicians such as John Conolly demonstrated the 'moral management' (ibid.: 78) of women in Victorian asylums. According to Showalter, women patients were encouraged to pursue domestic tasks mirroring those outside the asylum. If women steered away from lady-like behaviour, they were punished, as Showalter describes: 'At Colney Hatch, they were sedated, given cold baths, and secluded in padded cells, up to five times as frequently as male patients' (ibid.: 81).

The moral management of women patients was also extended to their appearance. Showalter states that the Victorian psychiatrists were greatly concerned with the appearance of women patients who were always highly commended if they showed interest in wearing pretty clothes or decorating their hair. Showalter shows how Granville's 1877 book, *Care and Cure of the Insane*, summed up these concerns: 'Dress is women's weakness, and in the treatment of lunacy it should be an instrument of control, and therefore recovery'. On the other hand, Showalter states that women who paid too much attention to their appearance were also considered insane. A photograph, for example, taken by medical director James Crichton Browne, portrays a female asylum patient believed to be displaying 'intense vanity'. She is heavily decorated in leaves and jewellery with dress that may be considered as unsuitable for her age. These treatments designed to keep femininity intact and female behaviour under control were indicative of life within the Victorian asylum for women. I shall now turn to Showalter's chapter on psychiatric modernism.

Showalter goes on to argue that the second generation of nineteenth-century psychiatrists was influenced by Darwinian ideas about sexual difference. Darwin suggested in his 1871 work, *The Descent of Man*, that through natural selection men would excel over women in the disciplines of art, philosophy and science because of their naturally higher levels of energy, courage and so forth. Darwin proposed that although women possessed characteristics including intuition and perception, these were associated with the lower races and were therefore signs of inferiority. Such ideas influenced how men and women were perceived in terms of their mental state. Women were seen to possess less energy as it was exhausted by their reproductive capacities. Therefore, their cells were seen as passive and depleted, whereas men's cells were seen as energetic. Women were also seen as naturally inclined to look after children and their husbands. They were also considered to pass on insanity to their female children; Showalter describes how Darwinian psychiatrists agreed that this was seen as an explanation for the greater numbers of women within asylums.

Moving on to the twentieth century, Showalter states that the postwar period brought a new female malady, that of schizophrenia. According to Showalter, literary texts such as Marguerite Sechaye's *Autobiography of a Schizophrenic Girl* represented the female schizophrenic as 'the symbol of linguistic, religious, and sexual breakdown and rebellion' (ibid.: 204). The treatments for schizophrenia, which included ECT, lobotomy and insulin shock (see Chapter 3), were given more to women than to men. She argues that statistical evidence reveals that women receiving ECT exceeded male patients by as much as a ratio of two or three to one. She suggests that representations of ECT found in film and photography generally reflect male power and female submission. The patient about to receive ECT is always presented as female. She is portrayed as passively laid out with a peaceful expression on her face. Showalter states that the patient is always feminised, be they male or female, and the doctor giving the ECT is always presented as male.

The surgical procedure of lobotomy, whereby parts of the brain tissue are severed, has also been given more to women than men as a cure for madness. Since 1941 the majority of the 15,000 lobotomies performed in England have been on women. A well-recommended psychiatric textbook of the 1970s, suggests a lobotomy to help a woman stay within a marriage to an unsuitable husband when medication has failed to work, and when separation is impossible due to religious beliefs or financial and emotional dependence upon the husband.

Showalter suggests that the treatment of insulin shock also held connotations for encouraging acceptable female behaviour. The women nurses administered the insulin and the patients were then put to bed to await the impending coma. According to Showalter, this represents the nurse as playing a maternal role and encourages infantile regression on the part of the female patient. This was also actively encouraged using additional treatments such as regular hot baths and a diet of sugar and starch.

There was an extensive body of English literature produced by women between the 1920s and the early 1960s, containing narratives that discuss madness, institutionalisation and ECT. Through the metaphor of schizophrenia, Showalter suggests, women were making statements about their cultural situation. Schizophrenia represented female rebellion and a break away from conforming within the feminine role. According to Showalter, the treatments for schizophrenia can be transformed 'into symbolic episodes of punishment for intellectual ambition, domestic defiance, and sexual autonomy' (ibid.: 210).

## Psychosurgery as violence

I will now turn to a 1987 study by Diane Hudson, a mental health practitioner, who examines the connections between psychosurgery, women and the female role. Hudson states that the psychosurgical technique of leucotomy (previously named as lobotomy) involves destroying brain tissue using a variety of procedures. Inserting hot wires and radioactive 'seeds' can destroy the brain tissue. Hudson cites the 'free hand' (Hudson 1987: 112) procedure involving placing a scalpel through a hole in the skull and severing brain tissue, as a favoured technique within psychiatry. This psychiatric procedure was widely used in the treatment of schizophrenia up to the 1960s.

Currently it is used less frequently and is limited for the treatment of intractable depression and obsessive-compulsive disorder. A psychiatric text, intended for training psychiatrists, states that there are twenty to thirty psychosurgical operations every year. These will only be performed if all other psychiatric treatments, such as medication and psychological treatments, have been exhausted. The text indicates that modern technology has meant that the procedure is now less crude: 'The older "blind" operations have been replaced by stereotactic procedures that allow the lesions to be placed more accurately' (Gelder *et al.* 2001: 176). Analysis of gender difference with regards to leucotomies is not outlined in this text although this has been documented, as we have seen, by Showalter.

Hudson identifies a relationship between psychosurgery and attempts to control women's behaviour. In the attempt to obtain statistical information about leucotomy, she found that since psychosurgical procedures began in 1888, more women than men had received them. Hudson suggests that the predominance of women patients receiving leucotomy has its roots in psychiatry's emphasis upon considering that psychiatric symptoms result from biological causes. It is thought that women's bodies are more prone to biological defects because of their hormones and reproductive capacities: 'Psychiatry is increasingly becoming biologically determinist, particularly with regard to women' (Hudson 1987: 115). Hudson states that this attitude involves attempts to remove the defect by controlling the individual's body, leaving their social environment unchanged. Invariably patients return to experience the social and emotional conditions that form the basis of their mental distress.

Psychosurgical procedures, in the form of leucotomy, are often suggested by mental health professionals for women whose behaviour is deemed undesirable by the people in their lives, including husbands and relatives. Hudson's study involves seven women who have attended a psychiatric rehabilitation day centre for over ten years. These women had been treated with leucotomy to address various behaviours. These women had been the victims of violent behaviour directed towards them by men encountered in their lives and had, not surprisingly, reacted to their predicament by becoming distressed. However, these reactions were considered as mental illnesses within the mental health system for which women were given leucotomies as a means, in effect, of curbing their undesirable responses and behaviour.

Five of the seven leucotomised women in Hudson's study were diagnosed with depression. Of the other two, one was diagnosed as schizophrenic and the other as mentally handicapped or having a learning disability. The causative factors behind the women's depression were identified by mental health practitioners as 'learned helplessness', 'manipulative behaviour', and the 'inability to arouse sympathy without arousing aversion'. Hudson found, however, that the factors behind the depression were due to the women's experiences of sexual and physical abuse from men encountered in their lives that were ignored by the psychiatric profession. Some had been sexually and physically abused by their fathers or husbands, others raped by strangers. In response to such experiences, many of these women became depressed.

Four of the women in Hudson's study, two married and two unmarried, were diagnosed as depressed as it was considered that they were unable to form 'normal' relationships with men. One of these women had experienced mental cruelty from her husband; another had sustained broken bones from physical abuse from her husband spanning several years. Hudson states how leucotomy was suggested for each of these women to help them remain within the confines of their marital relationships. The two unmarried women had both experienced sexual abuse as children. Their male social workers suggested they have a leucotomy to lessen their 'abnormal distrust of men' (ibid.: 118). Hudson describes how another woman's life had previously centred on her husband and family. The violence that ensued caused her to feel depressed, that her life was meaningless. Several women became opposed to resuming intimate relationships with men, and some had reacted to violence by displaying confrontational behaviour.

Hudson states how these different responses to violence were interpreted by the mental health system as evidence of mental illness. Attempts to avoid confrontation were portrayed as demonstrating apathy and passivity and labelled as depression. The women who confronted their aggressors were perceived as having hostile and aggressive personas and, in these cases, the label of personality disorder was attributed. Hudson states that when women presented these ways of reacting to violence, 'little or no attempt was made by the psychiatric professionals to take account of the causative factors in women's lives' (ibid.: 110).

## Reconsidering psychiatry as patriarchal oppression

Radical feminists identify oppressive patriarchal systems that reinforce popular conceptions of women as passive and submissive, and control the female body and sexuality. Both Showalter and Hudson identify psychiatry as being indicative of such a system. Showalter reveals how historically, perceptions about correct and respectable female behaviour have been reflected in cultural images of mad women, and have influenced their diagnosis and treatment. A Foucauldian analysis can be applied to these ideas, whereby the female body can be considered as the site upon which prevailing ideas, or rather discourses, are inscribed. These are depicted, as Showalter reveals, in artistic and literary forms. These discourses then construct the ways in which the bodies of women are perceived within mental health practice. Showalter also identifies psychiatry as being concerned with correcting unfeminine, wayward behaviour by often-barbaric treatments. Hudson shows how the psychiatric procedure of leucotomy has been used to silence women when their behaviour is deemed unfeminine.

Such critiques, however, reveal hostility to any kind of mental health treatment that may also include psychological treatments that may benefit women. Anti-psychotic medications, for example, can reduce distressing psychotic symptoms such as hearing voices. Women can also be offered psychological treatments such as counselling or Cognitive Behavioural Therapy within mainstream mental health practice. The critiques offered by those who identify psychiatry as a wholly oppressive system are also in danger of suggesting that women patients in their various forms of mental distress are offering a conscious political statement against male authority. The celebration of the madwoman's seemingly rebellious social stance fails to consider that the lived experience of mental distress is hardly celebratory.

## Conclusion

In this chapter, I have outlined how feminists have theorised the body and women's oppression and how these theories have, in turn, been applied to understanding women's mental distress and its psychiatric treatment. Marxist and socialist feminists have highlighted the physical work done by women in their roles as mothers and carers, and how this contributes to their experiences of mental distress. Radical feminists have highlighted how patriarchal structures have controlled and regulated the female body and sexuality. Showalter and Hudson have applied this to psychiatry in their analysis of the ways in which female biology has been considered as responsible for women's mental distress. The female body, sexuality and behaviour have also been controlled by psychiatric practices including ECT, leucotomy operations and medication, which is highlighted by the greater numbers of women over men, being given these treatments.

As we will see, aspects of the theories espoused by feminists and other writers on women's distress outlined in this chapter can be applied to the experiences of women patients today. Although there have been changes in terms of women's economic position. Women of working age, for instance, in the UK, are generally less economically dependent on men. Yet, despite women's apparent liberation and independence from men, single women are consistently discussed in the press in a derogatory manner as sexual predators or binge drinkers. Single men hardly get a mention despite the fact that the number of single men has doubled over the past two decades. Along with factors such as unemployment and social isolation, male singledom is considered to contribute towards the increase in suicide rates among young men. They are three times more likely than women to kill themselves. The cause of this phenomenon are still debatable, but is it that twenty years ago men had a much clearer sense of who they were in terms of their roles? Did men feel better when it was undoubtedly the case that they were breadwinners? What effect has the blurring of gender roles had upon male embodiment? Do men feel squashed and invisible? Yet, at a time when gender roles were much more defined and distinct, women often felt belittled and oppressed in their presumed roles as mothers and homemakers, as the above perspectives demonstrate.

As I have stated, I do not address these questions regarding the effects of mental health diagnosis and treatment on male embodiment in this book. My focus upon the mental distress of women will now proceed through to the next chapter, where I outline historical notions of hysteria, which is the Latin word for uterus. I will then discuss some of the female hysterics who – depending upon your opinion – were fortunate enough to have Freud 'listen' to the often-obscure language of their bodies. The women presented in Freud and Breuer's *Studies on Hysteria* in 1895 were also fortunate enough to have someone acknowledge their desire for passion and the ways in which this was denied and unacknowledged in their social circumstances. This was as 'feminist' as Freud got. Thirty years later he made a statement that absolutely lacks any recognition of female sexual desire. Women, he said, in order to achieve sexual maturity, would have to give up their masculine clitoris for the 'truly' feminine vagina as the *central* focus of their sexual pleasure.

# Chapter 5

# Unspoken distress

As a mental health nurse in the community, I worked with a depressed young man whose body seemed to communicate something about him. He complained almost constantly of flu symptoms. His legs, he told me, felt like dead weights. Sometimes they felt so rooted to the ground that he felt he couldn't walk. He had a sense that his body was being dragged backwards, and he was full of aches and pains. When this man began to feel better through receiving psychological interventions where he began to speak in great detail about his painful relationship with both his parents, these symptoms gradually disappeared. He described how he felt his parents were always trying to hold him back and would not let him move forward in his life. It was as if his mind was using his body to tell the story of his experiences. Physical symptoms like these, which have no apparent medical cause, are generally referred to as conversion symptoms, or, less commonly, as 'hysteria'. The person presenting them often denies that there is any psychological connection to them.

This is what Freud encountered in his predominantly female patients that he wrote about in 1895, who presented to him a wide range of bodily symptoms. Rather than just 'looking' at these symptoms, he listened to them as a kind of language of the body and attached meanings to them in terms of what the women had experienced. Along the way, he devised a dynamic understanding of how painful feelings become, or are expressed as, painful bodily symptoms. He reports that these symptoms are, of course, real to the person presenting them, but something else is going on. Freud, of course, was a scientist. As a student at the University of Vienna in 1874, Sigmund Freud described himself to a friend as a 'godless medical student and an empiricist' (Freud in Gay 1988: 29). However, he felt rejected by, and began to separate from, the medical establishment with his interest in the origins of hysteria following his visit to Paris to study with the French physician Jean Martin Charcot, as we shall see.

Continuing to use a historical approach in the presentation of theory, I shall begin this chapter by outlining notions of the body in fifth-century BC Greek thought and how these influenced subsequent medical and cultural perceptions of hysteria, or more specifically, the 'wandering womb'. I will then discuss Freud and Breuer's understanding of hysteria and how this marked a radical shift away from preceding notions of this phenomenon. I then proceed to discuss Freud's fascinating notions of the relationship between the body and psychical processes. He rarely diverted from his discussion of the body and this is evident in his early writings on hysteria through to his writings on femininity and his notion of 'penis envy'.

The idea that women were inherently envious of penises provoked feminist thinkers, including Kate Millett, to accuse Freud of being a biological determinist. Although I agree with this accusation to some extent – especially in relation to Freud's ideas about the 'masculine' clitoris and the girl's necessary move towards her 'truly' feminine vagina – I nevertheless think that his early accounts of female hysterics are rather 'feminist', as I will try to demonstrate in this chapter. I also wish to emphasise that Freud's work is relevant to an understanding of the body and mental illness as he proposes that symptoms have specific meanings for the lived experience of the individual and do not merely relate a specific diagnosis of mental illness. He also contends that the body is a site of non-verbal communication, and focuses upon the importance of the correlations between psychical and physical processes in early development.

## The body in fifth-century BC Greece

Since the Enlightenment in the seventeenth century, scientific investigation has perceived the body as a system consisting of various organs that create a discrete biological and psychological entity. Most psychiatrists see psychiatric disorders such as depression or schizophrenia as resulting from a chemical imbalance in the brain. Similarly, emotion is something connected to neurological processes situated in the head.

In fifth-century BC Greece, however, perceptions of the self and the body appear to be vastly different from contemporary thought. The fifth-century BC Greek term for 'innards' was *splanchma*, which were thought to consist of the gallbladder, heart, lungs, blood vessels and liver. For the Greeks, these innards felt emotions such as grief, pity and love. Emotion was, therefore, considered to emerge from within the body and was not connected to a 'mind' situated in the brain. The source of consciousness was, therefore, not in the head but within the body. Additionally, the functions of bodily organs were determined, not by inner physiological processes, but by external deities. As Ruth Padel states, external forces such as wind, rain, sunshine and so forth, were perceived as filling the internal organs with disease or emotion: 'Changes of habit, such as change in the color of the wine you drink, cause changes, maybe dangerous ones, in the body. Changing winds cause disease . . . outside terrain causes inner disease' (1995: 9).

The fifth-century BC Greeks considered that swelling or movement of internal organs symbolised negativity and disease within the body. Inner movement occurred in reaction to passion or madness that was uncontrollable and diseased. Padel states that the negative connotations with wandering were gendered, as they were associated with the female body in the image of the 'wandering womb'. The womb, like all the innards, was considered to have a proper place within the body. When the womb was diseased and damaged it was considered to move around the body uncontrollably. Plato's *Timaeus*, for example, states that the womb 'left unfertilised long beyond the normal time, causes extreme unrest, strays about the body' and 'causes acute distress and disorders of all kinds' (1977: 123). This image of the wandering womb suggests that the womb, and therefore female sexuality, was beyond the control of external forces and gods. Perceived as having a life of its own, the womb was considered to wander causing harm within the body. The female body and female sexuality thus became synonymous with disease and badness.

## Hysteria: Greece and beyond

I will now provide an account of changes in constructions and in the treatment of hysteria starting with the Greeks, and discuss ways in which hysteria has been associated with women's bodies. Hippocrates coined the term 'hysteria', after the Greek word for uterus. In writings such as *Sicknesses of Women*, he describes the uterus as uncontrollable, moving at random around the body causing hysterical symptoms such as aches and pains, twitches, loss of speech and breathing difficulties. Aretaeus, the Cappadocian in the second century BC, maintains this image of the wandering womb but added animalistic references stating that the womb, or rather the 'female viscus', closely resembled an animal (Aretaeus in Slavney 1990: 13).

Galen, a near contemporary of Aretaeus, stated that dissection of the female body proved that the uterus was, in fact, a stationary organ and put forward the suggestion that hysteria occurred as a result of abnormal sexual functioning. Hysteria was considered to particularly affect widows and a remedy was believed to be marriage and pregnancy. The perceived links between hysterical symptoms and uterine causes remained unchallenged into the seventeenth century. In a 1603 monograph of Edward Jorden entitled *A Brief Discourse of a Disease Called The Suffocation of the Mother*, both external and internal factors are considered to affect the uterus. Once diseased, and upon making contact with other bodily organs, the uterus could produce a wide range of illnesses such as chorea, paralysis, suffocation and coma.

Although considerations of the links between the uterus and hysteria are explicit in the writings of Jorden, a decline in these beliefs had begun during this period. This was characterised by awareness of the fact that symptoms of hysteria frequently occurred in men as well as women. However, as men do not possess a uterus, it was thought that their spleens were responsible for producing symptoms that were termed hypochondriasis rather than hysteria.

Despite attempts to dispel beliefs that the uterus was solely responsible for the symptoms of hysteria, physicians failed to explain the greater occurrences of these symptoms in women. The physician Thomas Willis attempted to provide explanations by suggesting that the female brain and nervous system were weaker than the male's. Thus, emotions such as fear and sadness would affect women more profoundly, increasing the potential for hysterical symptoms.

Through the eighteenth and nineteenth centuries hysteria continued to be linked to the nervous system and to women. Various writings of the period indicate the perceived connections between hysteria and women, and moralistic attempts to control what was considered as the erratic nature of womanhood. Henry Maudsley, for example, said of hysterics in 1879:

> that their perverted moral state is somehow connected with the action of the reproductive organs on an unstable nervous system seems probable because it is mostly met in unmarried women, is prone to exhibit erotic features, and is sometimes cured by marriage.
>
> (Maudsley in Slavney 1990)

Alternative treatments of hysteria were practised in the eighteenth and early nineteenth centuries by animal magnetism, mesmerism and hypnotism to provide a background to the work of Jean-Martin Charcot and, subsequently, of Freud. Franz Anton Mesmer, a Viennese physician, was impressed by the recent discovery of the potential of electricity. He considered that an invisible 'universal fluid', that he thought to exist in the bodies of animals, was similar to the substance that gave magnets their power. Mesmer considered that various illnesses resulted from an imbalance in universal fluid and cure was to be found in connecting patients to the source of this fluid. In fact, Mesmer used a magnet in his experiments, which he considered as the most obvious instrument to connect his patients to astral forces. Such experiments consisted of large water-filled covered tubs, which also contained magnetised iron filings. Mesmer's patients would stand in the tubs, which had iron rods projected through the lids. His patients were asked to position the rods towards the affected areas of their bodies. As Michael H. Stone states, Mesmer dressed up in a purple robe, looking like a magician, and set about inducing a 'hysteric crisis' (1997: 59). The patients, who were mostly women, would subsequently fall into a trance or deep sleep and would apparently awake completely healed. There is thus a focus here on treatment of the body in order to treat disease. This practice is not unlike some of the physical therapies such as ECT and insulin coma introduced in the 1930s and 1940s.

Magnetism was an elaborate physical intervention and, like ECT for example, it was unknown how it actually worked. These treatments are also highly theatrical and focused upon the charismatic power of the central figure of the doctor who conducted the procedure. Magnetism is also similar to ECT and insulin coma as the recipient is passive. The procedure of magnetism fell into disrepute in the late eighteenth century when it was investigated by the royal commission of Louis XVI. However, occasionally, followers of Mesmer, named as mesmerists, continued to practise in Europe and the British Isles, although it was greatly opposed in many established hospitals and mesmerists were forced to practise secretly.

James Braid, a Scottish physician, became interested in the phenomenon of mesmeric sleep following attendance at seances organised by a travelling mesmerist. Braid subsequently studied artificially induced sleep and devised a new vocabulary of concepts such as neuro-hypnotism and hypnotism. Braid attempted to separate hypnotism from earlier practices of mesmerism and stated that hypnotism was brought about by an impression upon the nervous system that did not involve any unproven mystical factors. Braid was among the first to distinguish between functional and organic diseases, and emphasised the way in which functional disorders could be aided by suggestion through hypnosis.

Although Braid never found acceptance for his ideas in England, the French physician Charcot revived hypnosis in Paris in 1878. Charcot worked with hysterics and gave lectures on the condition at his clinic in the Paris hospital La Salpêtrière, gaining enormous popularity from all over the world. He defined hysteria either as a condition caused by a traumatic injury in the central nervous system or by a defect acquired hereditarily. Charcot also emphasised the role of the emotions in the production of hysterical symptoms, which, of course, was to be later developed by Freud. Charcot considered that a capacity to be hypnotised is, in itself, characteristic of hysteria.

Charot stated, unlike many of his predecessors, that the symptoms of hysteria could be found in both men and women, and suggested that the link between hysteria and the uterus did not exist:

> Keep it well in mind and this should not require a great effort, that the word 'hysteria' means nothing, and little by little you will acquire the habit of speaking of hysteria in man without thinking in any way of the uterus.
>
> (Charcot in Veith 1965: 232)

At the Salpêtrière, there were facilities for male victims of railway accidents. However, as it was a hospital for women, most of Charcot's patients were female. The representation of these women in photography became the main focus of his work.

The often-startling photographs of these hysterics have been made into three volumes entitled *Iconographie photographique de la Salpêtrière*. One of the photographs depicts fifteen-year-old Augustine. She exhibited a range of hysterical symptoms including imitations and enactments from silent films and nineteenth-century paintings (such as Millais' *Ophelia*) and seeing things in black and white. She rebelled against the hospital regime with outbursts of anger and violence for which she was anaesthetised with ether or chloroform, and placed in a locked cell. She managed to escape the hospital by disguising herself as a man. Nobody who tried was able to subsequently locate her.

Although Charcot appeared to resist emphasising connections between hysteria and the uterus, he nevertheless focused upon the female body in demonstrating hysterical symptoms. He considered that the ovaries and the breasts were particularly sensitive 'hysterogenic zones'. This led to the invention of an 'ovary compressor' to initiate and stop hysterical attacks. The ovarian area of the female body, when pressed, seemed to produce hysterical convulsions.

Elaine Showalter states that, although Charcot insisted that hysteria could be present in both sexes, 'both he and his staff repeatedly fell back on stereotypes that equated it with the female personality' (1998: 34). For instance, hysterics were frequently described as possessing intense vanity. The lectures that Charcot directed in a large amphitheatre at the Salpêtrière involved hysterical women being hypnotised by his students, who were mostly men. Many of these women became showpieces admired by audiences of intellectual and bohemian society, and the photographic representations of these lectures became widely used in nineteenth-century psychiatric practice.

Freud considered the practice of hypnosis as legitimate and this initiated him, during the years of 1885 and 1886, to study with Charcot at the Salpêtrière hospital in Paris. Freud became intrigued by Charcot's work and was particularly impressed by the way in which he initiated and stopped hysterical attacks by hypnosis. This influenced Freud's subsequent work with his hysterical female patients in Vienna. As Showalter suggests, of the many admirers of Charcot, it was Freud who possessed the 'charisma and determination to build up a theoretical empire' (ibid.: 38).

Freud's early work with hysterics consisted of dealing with symptoms such as coughs, headaches and muteness. Freud and his colleague, Joseph Breuer, proposed that, rather than stemming from traumatic injury or hereditary factors, hysteria can occur in both men and women. They suggested hysteria could be due to trauma occurring in a daydream or other distracted state, with the trauma, absent from consciousness, being converted into bodily symptoms. Through the practice of hypnosis, Freud and Breuer proposed that the original trauma would resurface so that the hysterical symptoms would disappear.

## Breuer and Anna 'O'

Particularly important in this was Breuer's discoveries with his patient Bertha Pappenheim, or Anna 'O', who was treated by him between 1880 and 1882. Anna was a twenty-one-year-old Viennese woman. Breuer described her as 'markedly intelligent, with an astonishingly quick grasp of things and penetrating intuition' (Freud and Breuer 1895: 21) According to Breuer, Anna was expected by her family to complete her schooling by the age of sixteen and she subsequently had no outlet for her intelligence. As a daughter within a middle-class Jewish family, Anna was expected to pursue a life of domesticity. Her brother however, although less intelligent, went to university. As a compensation for her lack of intellectual stimulation, Anna would frequently resort to daydreaming, which she described as her 'private theatre' (ibid.: 22).

Part of Anna's expected role within her household was to look after her father suffering from tuberculosis, who contracted an infection that took his life in 1880. Following his death, her hysterical symptoms began. They included headache, a severe cough, paralyses, muscular rigidity, refusal of food, hallucinations and insomnia. Anna also experienced speech difficulties whereby she appeared to not understand her native German, but communicated only in English. When asked to read aloud in French or Italian, although fluent in these languages, she would only produce English translations. Anna's speech transformed into confusing utterances consisting of the five languages in which she had been educated.

Breuer developed a method of treatment whereby he asked Anna to relate to him her fantasies and thoughts, which she later named as the 'talking cure'. These utterances brought out randomly or under hypnosis, consisted of recollections of events that had occurred while Anna was caring for her sick father. These episodes had occurred while she was in an emotionally heightened or depressed, distracted state. In the course of time, as Anna was able to recall and verbalise the original trauma, her hysterical symptoms disappeared. According to Breuer these traumatic events had been repressed and had symbolically surfaced as hysterical symptoms manifested in Anna's body.

There are examples of Breuer's ability to relate Anna's hysterical symptoms to an earlier traumatic event. Anna's persistent cough had originally occurred as she sat by her father's bedside, and had heard the sound of dancing music coming from a neighbour's house. Anna had a sudden desire to be at this gathering and to be part of the celebrations, but was overcome with guilt. Since this event, as Breuer states, 'she reacted to any markedly rhythmical music with a *tussis nervosa*' (ibid.: 30) (or nervous cough).

Another example concerned Anna's hysterical symptom of a rigid right arm. Breuer encouraged Anna to recall under hypnosis the occasion when it first began. Her mother, although sharing the responsibility of caring for Anna's father, had gone away for a short period and Anna had woken up in an anxious state about her feverish father. Anna was awaiting the arrival of a surgeon who was due to operate on him. While sitting at his bedside, Anna had her right arm positioned over the back of the chair. She had fallen into a waking dream and saw a black snake approaching her father trying to bite him. As she attempted to fend off the snake, she found her right arm was paralysed. The snake vanished and Anna tried to pray but could find no words to express her feelings in her native German. However, she was able to recall and verbalise English children's verses. The waking dream ended with the approach of a whistling train carrying the surgeon.

At the end of his treatment of Anna, Breuer attempted to reproduce this hallucination by arranging the room in which he treated her to resemble her father's sick room. With Breuer's help, Anna recollected the hallucination of the snake and was able to speak in German, whereas, when the hallucination occurred originally, she was only able to pray in English. Consequently, as Breuer describes, by reproducing the original trauma Anna became free from disturbances she had previously expressed.

The treatment of Anna ended abruptly when she imagined she was giving birth to Breuer's child. In response, Breuer terminated the treatment. Freud was eager to hear more about the case of Anna 'O' from Breuer, on his return from the Salpêtrière where he had studied with Charcot. Freud identified Anna's hysterical pregnancy as transference whereby the patient transfers his or her emotions to the analyst. Often the analyst can represent a parental figure. Thus, according to Freud, Anna's transference feelings to Breuer masked her desire for her father. Freud proceeded to specify sexuality as being the source of hysterical complaints. By 1897, Freud had abandoned the concept that hysteria is caused by an earlier sexual trauma usually initiated by fathers, which Ernest Jones named as the 'seduction theory', which I will discuss below. Alternatively, Freud proposed that these early traumas were, in fact, fantasies. Thus, women were fantasising seduction by their fathers. This marks the beginnings of Freud's concepts of femininity, the Oedipus complex and infantile sexuality that I will also discuss below.

## Breuer and Anna 'O': feminist interpretations

The case of Anna 'O' has provoked much discussion among feminist writers. Rather than considering the term hysteria to be derogatory, such writers suggest that the presentation of hysterical symptoms symbolises the female voice and resistance to patriarchal oppression. Showalter, for example, has stated that, for Breuer, Anna's hysteria was an escape from her ties to a life of domesticity set by her family. Breuer clearly considers how her lack of intellectual activity 'left her with an unemployed surplus of mental liveliness and energy, and this found an outlet in the constant activity of her imagination' (ibid.: 41). Showalter states that it is clear that Breuer respected the liveliness and intelligence of his patient. By receptively listening to her and being attentive to ways in which her bodily symptoms symbolised repressed psychical conflict, Breuer was able to enter, as Showalter describes, 'a female world of consciousness repressed by the patriarchal structure, the world of the unconscious' (Showalter 1985: 157).

Dianne Hunter focuses upon Anna 'O's loss of speech and childlike babble and considers how it suggests the ways in which she resented her position within her family and thus refused to speak and acknowledge the patriarchal language of the world surrounding her. Drawing upon the work of Lacan (which I will discuss in the next chapter), Hunter states 'the power to formulate sentences coincides developmentally with a recognition of the power of the father' (Hunter 1983: 474). Anna's rejection of speech and subsequent babble could represent a rejection of the cultural values of her upbringing and a return to the pre-Oedipal, maternal space occupied by the infant before language. According to Hunter, hysteria is a means of expressing what cannot be stated verbally due to the surrounding social conditions imposing patriarchal values, and a 'feminine discourse in which the body signifies what social conditions make it impossible to state linguistically' (ibid.: 485). Symptoms such as '*globus hystericus*' (difficulty in swallowing) can be seen to represent the physically blocked words of women within patriarchal culture.

Breuer's analysis of Anna 'O' highlights how women's non-verbal means of communication can be acknowledged and valued. Breuer was able to focus upon Anna's lived experience. He identified her surrounding oppressive situation whereby she was not allowed to proceed with her education and was tied to a life of domesticity. This, in turn, stunted her creativity whereby the only outlet for her intelligence was through daydreaming.

The case of Anna 'O' written by Breuer, and four further case studies written by Freud, were collected together in the form of *Studies on Hysteria* (1895). Breuer focused upon the surrounding social conditions of women patients as he demonstrated in the case of Anna 'O'. This is also evident in Freud's remaining four case studies, although it is clear that Freud was increasingly keen to attach sexual meanings to hysterical symptoms, which was clearly necessary for the formation of his theories about the Oedipus complex and infantile sexuality. Focus upon sexuality unfortunately took precedence over women's social position in Freud's analysis of Dora (which I will discuss briefly following his other case studies). His writings following his focus upon hysteria with regards to women and their bodies, which he largely undertook almost thirty years later, are rather disappointing. However, Freud's writings on the body demonstrate his commitment to exploring and highlighting the correlations between the mind and body, as I will now demonstrate.

## Freud on the body, femininity and women's mental distress

Elizabeth Grosz in her paper, 'Psychoanalysis and the Body' (in Price and Shildrick 1999), states that psychoanalytic theory appears on the surface as opposed to the body with its emphasis on analysis and interpretation of the workings of the mind. Perhaps surprisingly then, from his early pre-psychoanalytic writings, Freud focuses a great deal on the body and this aspect of his work has been largely unrecognised. *Project for a Scientific Psychology* in 1895, for example, reveals his endeavour to find correlations between neurophysiological and psychical processes. Freud's early writings on hysteria such as *Studies on Hysteria* in 1895 and *The Aetiology of Hysteria* in 1896, reveal his concepts of the way in which trauma is repressed by psychical processes and translated into non-verbal bodily symptoms.

## 'Joining in the conversation': the body and hysteria

In these various case studies presented in *Studies on Hysteria*, the divergence between Freud and Breuer emerges. As I discussed above, Breuer states that trauma resurfacing when the patient is in a daydream or distracted state, lies behind the development of hysterical symptoms. He also emphasises the importance of the technique of hypnosis in bringing back the original trauma to consciousness. In the remaining four case studies, Freud introduces several concepts that reveal his divergence from Breuer and which also emphasise his letting go of hypnosis as a method in the treatment of hysterical symptoms. As I have stated, Freud's major divergence from Breuer is his introduction of the importance of sexuality in the aetiology of hysteria. Freud's considerations of the hysterical body, as Monique David-Menard points out, suggest, 'Hysterical symptoms and crises constitute a pantomime of sexual pleasure' (1989: 3).

Through focusing on the symptoms of hysteria manifest in the bodies of his female patients, Freud formulates many of his psychoanalytic theories including conversion, defence, regression and neurosis as conflict between the ego and libido. According to Freud, the libido is an energy or drive that is sexual in nature. I think it is useful to understand the libido as a life instinct or drive, rather than a constant desire to have sex. Revealing his interest in the correlations between the mind and body, Freud seems to imply that the libido exists on the borderline between the body and mind. It is also subject to discharge. This process is described in Freud's theory of conversion whereby psychical conflict is transferred into somatic symptoms such as paralyses and pains.

Freud states that an idea can be repressed because of its unacceptable or intolerable content. Repression is perhaps like swallowing something down so that it seems to have gone, but in actual fact it is still with us. It remains undigested. In Freud's estimation, the idea then has an excess of libidinal energy attached to it because although 'forgotten', it is still 'alive' and represents what once was very significant. In Freud's estimation, this libidinal energy becomes detached from the repressed idea and is transformed into innervational energy. Freud thus reveals how certain parts of the body can become libidinally cathected into what he describes as erotogenic or hysterogenic zones. The body thereby becomes a symbol of that which cannot be tolerated psychically or translated through words, as Pontalis and Laplanche explain: 'what specifies conversion symptoms is their symbolic meaning: they express repressed ideas through the medium of the body' (Laplanche and Pontalis 1988: 90). An example of this process is revealed in Freud's case study of Fraulein Elizabeth von R.

Freud undertook the treatment of Elizabeth von R. in 1892. She complained of pains in her legs and difficulty in walking. As stated, Freud was increasingly formulating his central notion that sexual life is rather important. Consequently he considered that Elizabeth's symptoms were indeed sexual in origin. When carrying out a physical examination, Freud pinched Elizabeth's thighs and her face revealed a sensation of pleasure rather than pain. As Freud describes, 'She cried out – and I could not help thinking, as with a voluptuous tickling – her face flushed, she threw back her head, closed her eyes, her trunk bent backwards' (Freud and Breuer 1895: 137). Freud realised that he had touched a hysterogenic zone; the concealed sexual desire behind the pain was aroused in Elizabeth by the stimulation of the body parts associated with these thoughts.

Freud presents Elizabeth's life as being a series of unfortunate episodes. She nursed her father who later died. One of her sisters married and alienated herself from her family, another sister died during pregnancy, a brother-in-law exhibited difficult behaviour affecting the rest of the family, and Elizabeth's mother suffered from a serious illness. Although these experiences were obviously traumatic, Freud could not identify one that appeared to precipitate Elizabeth's hysterical symptoms in her legs. Freud tried hypnosis but Elizabeth refused to submit. Similarly, at this time Freud also encountered other patients including Miss Lucy R., who also refused the hypnotic technique. Freud began to consider that the patient, in fact, knew everything that was of significance to their symptoms and that it was only a question of enabling them to communicate it.

At first Freud tried the pressure technique whereby he would place his hands on the patient's forehead while telling them that they could remember everything. However, Freud found that asking the patient to say anything that came into her head irrespective of its irrelevance, was a successful technique which he used with Elizabeth von R. This technique, which was later to become known as 'free association', was a laborious exercise. There were long silences during which Freud asked Elizabeth what she was thinking to which she would reply that she had no thoughts at all. This was the beginnings of Freud's discovery and theory of resistance, as Peter Gay states: 'Freud was learning about resistance. It was resistance that kept Elizabeth von R. from talking; it was her wilful forgetting, he thought, that had produced her conversion symptoms in the first place' (Gay 1988: 71).

Freud concluded that Elizabeth had fended off desire for her brother-in-law and death wishes towards her dying sister. Her bodily symptoms symbolised her conflict between being pressured to nurse her sick father and her erotic desires for her brother-in-law. These bodily symptoms flared up during the start of the analysis. Freud would provoke a memory whereby Elizabeth would feel sudden pain that would intensify when she began to relate to him the necessary details. The pain would then disappear once Elizabeth had fully communicated these facts. Freud stated that Elizabeth's painful legs 'began to "join in the conversation" during our analyses' (Freud and Breuer 1895: 148). He considered that Elizabeth was not revealing the whole story and insisted that her pains had to be talked away.

Freud eventually made clear his suggestion of her desire for her brother-in-law, which was met with resistance: 'She complained at this moment of the most frightful pains, and made one last desperate effort to reject the explanation' (ibid.: 157). Elizabeth's pains subsided fully once she finally became conscious of, and spoke about her sexual desires that were the origins of her hysterical bodily symptoms. She revealed that at her dying sister's bedside she had wished for her sister's death and at the same time a thought flashed through her mind about her shortly to be widowed brother-in-law: 'Now he is free again and I can be his wife' (ibid.: 156).

In his emphasis upon the bodily symptoms of hysteria, Freud argued that these symptoms are a result of repressed sexual desire. Elizabeth von R.'s body, which Freud described as joining in the conversation, acts as a symbol upon which hidden conflict is played out. The repressed idea is considered too unacceptable. It is then converted into painful, but more bearable physical symptoms. In his case studies, Freud revealed that bodily symptoms do not stem merely from a pathological source warranting a cure. He considered that they result from psychical conflict and experiences in the patient's life. Freud also focused upon the conflicts within women's lives. He revealed the conflict between women's ties to domesticity and their desires. His other case studies reveal similar themes. Miss Lucy R. for example, experiences conflict over sexual desire and rejection by her employer. Katharina's and Rosalia H.'s distress stem from experiences of incest and unwanted sexual advances. These women, through their bodies, present these conflicts and Freud interprets them. Furthermore, in *Studies on Hysteria*, Freud presented these individual women as named, actual subjects, not as objects.

Freud's perceptions of his women patients appear rather radical considering he presented them in 1895, when attention to and recognition of female sexual desire was rather limited. He acknowledged women's sexual desire and considered that women's domestic ties were often in conflict with their wishes not only for passion, but their desire to think. Modern day hysterical symptoms might have a radically different expression than those of Freud's patients, but he made clear that bodily symptoms, often corresponding to psychical and social conflict that cannot be translated into words, are worth attention. This approach does indeed differ from that espoused in mainstream mental health practice, which suggests that the body is merely a system of symptoms relating to a biological source. Freud certainly does acknowledge the lived experiences of his women patients. He thereby considers their distress in the context of their lives.

In the case of eighteen-year-old Dora in 1905, however, Freud seemed to ignore her concerns about her intellectual aspirations that were stifled by her family and social situation. Dora listened to Freud's interpretations of her hysteric symptoms, which included a choking, nausea and complete loss of voice. She told Freud that her father's friend Herr K. had made unwelcome sexual advances towards her by a lake. Dora's father suggested to Freud that she had made it all up. After all, as her father stated, she had been reading books on the physiology of love and had clearly become overexcited as a result (Freud 1905a: 26). Freud proposed that her choking and nausea were because of her feeling of disgust. This disgust, for Freud, was actually pleasure that had been transformed into a negative emotion. He suggested that her other hysterical symptoms were due to incestuous desires and bisexual wishes. After three months, with her hysteria intact, Dora said goodbye to Freud with good wishes for the new year and did not return, as Freud expected and movingly expressed, 'I knew Dora would not come back again' (ibid.: 109).

The case of Dora presents to some as a clear 'up yours' to Freud and his perceived sexist theories about women's bodies. Yet in reading his account, it is clear that he is sympathetic to Dora. As Janet Malcolm states in her essay on Dora in *The Purloined Clinic* (1992), Freud evokes a sense of sympathy in the reader because of his narrative powers. Malcolm states that Dora might well have invented the scene by the lake and many writers might suggest in their presentation of this account, that lying women are nothing but trouble for respectable men. Malcolm asserts that those who accuse Freud of a limited capacity for sympathy towards Dora, should consider that the sympathy aroused in them is a direct response to the 'artifacts of Freud's rhetoric' (1992: 26).

## The seduction theory: bodily violation

Freud's perception of bodily symptoms in hysteria as sexual in origin, continues in his essay, *The Aetiology of Hysteria* (1896). Here, Freud states that the hysteric's body communicates real traumatic experiences in early childhood. He states that hysterical symptoms result from a lived experience whereby the patient's body has been violated as the result of sexual abuse by an adult: 'At the bottom of every case of hysteria there are one or more occurrences of premature sexual experience' (1896: 203). Freud suggests that the particular experience of seduction determines the type of neurosis. In the case of obsessional neurosis for example, the sexual abuse is active or involves rape. In hysteria, the abuse is a passive sexual experience. Freud explains that the passive experience means that the abused child acts passively during it. Furthermore, Freud states that the abuse fails to produce a response in the individual because it occurs as a pre-sexual sexual event when the child is not capable of sexual emotions.

Freud states that it is not the trauma itself that produces the hysterical symptoms but, rather, the memory of the trauma which is triggered later during puberty. He writes: 'No hysterical symptom can arise from a real experience alone, but that in every case the memory of earlier experiences awakened in association to it plays a part in causing the symptom' (ibid.: 197). This trauma does not become repressed until a second event occurs which brings associations with the first event. The second event causes the individual to feel disgust at the excitations that the memory of the original event may bring. Freud suggests that the affect of this memory causes a surge of excitation that overwhelms the ego so that it cannot be translated into psychical terms but, rather, becomes repressed. Freud insisted that the repression is at first successful but then fails but does not enter consciousness. These excitations are, according to Freud, transformed into innervational energy, which is transported into parts of the body. The body thereby becomes a symbol of repressed libidinal ideas. Freud proposed, as he did in *Studies on Hysteria*, that through concentration upon the bodily symptoms of hysteria, repressed ideas could be unravelled, understood and verbalised.

By 1897, Freud had renounced his theory of seduction. In a letter to his friend Fliess in 1897 he wrote: 'I no longer believe in my *neurotica* (theory of the neuroses)' (Freud in Masson 1985: 264). He began to argue that the various accounts of seduction by fathers told by his women patients were, in fact, repressed fantasies. As Teresa Brennan states, 'what Freud abandoned was the idea that the sole cause of a psychoneurosis was an actual seduction' (1992: 29). Freud emphasised that the *effects* of real events were similar to fantasised ones. Whether or not the actual seduction had taken place, of importance was the way in which the individual dealt with it. If the idea or memory had been removed from consciousness, in other words if it had been repressed, it was this that gave rise to the hysterical symptom.

Freud did not abandon the seduction theory completely and did occasionally acknowledge its occurrence, for instance, in suggesting that child sexual abuse (although he never called it by this term) could play a part in the aetiology of neurosis. However, with his developing theories of infantile sexuality and what was later to be named as the 'Oedipus complex', Freud continued to emphasise the role of repression and fantasy. Thus, Freud's theory of the aetiology of hysteria changed from one in which sexuality is imposed on the infant's body from outside, to one which specifies that sexual desire emerges from the infant's body desiring real or fantasised seduction.

The reader might be interested at this stage to consider Freud's other writings on the body that predominantly relate to the neuroses. As I have stated, a large part of this book is dedicated to psychosis. However, two of the people (the women) I present as case studies in Chapter 8 experience 'neurotic' symptoms. Furthermore, Freud's writings on the body demonstrate his commitment to the correlations between the mind and body. I shall therefore continue.

## Infantile sexuality: body parts as erotogenic zones

In *Three Essays on the Theory of Sexuality* in 1905, Freud argued that sexual life begins in childhood. This was highly controversial at the time, and many people find this idea disturbing today. Freud proposed that parts of the infant's body become the objects to which it directs its sexual instincts; Freud called these objects erotogenic zones. In a footnote added in 1915, however, Freud specifies that any part of the body, both internal and external, can constitute an erotogenic zone: 'After further reflection and after taking other observations into account, I have been led to ascribe the quality of erotogenicity to all parts of the body and to all the internal organs' (1905b: 184). According to Freud, the infant's instincts and drives are innate. In order to develop psychically, and to establish its identity as autonomous and distinct, the infant has to pass through three phases of psychosexual development to which the instincts are directed. Freud characterises these phases as 'auto-erotic' whereby the infant finds the sexual object not in the external world but in its own body.

Freud states that up to around six months, the infant's libidinal energies are free flowing within its body and the infant has no concept of inside or outside. These energies then become blocked or redirected towards specific zones of the infant's body. Freud characterises the oral phase as the first stage of libidinal development. The mouth is the primary source of pleasure and this stage is associated with the sense of completeness and fulfilment the child gains through sucking and biting. The sexual instinct is first satisfied within an anaclitic relationship, usually with the mother's breast. Here the sexual aim corresponds with a vital need for nourishment: 'sexual activity has not yet been separated from the ingestion of food; nor are opposite currents within the activity differentiated' (ibid.: 198). However, Freud states the instinct then becomes autonomous and obtains pleasure from an auto-erotic source. Freud cites thumb sucking as an example of this. In this instance, the sexual instinct is not directed towards a vital object providing nourishment, but to one that provides sexual pleasure and serves to reflect this initial experience of satisfaction.

The anal phase, which according to Freud occurs approximately between the ages of two and four, refers to the way in which the infant proceeds to gain pleasure from withholding and expelling its faeces. Freud identifies the opposites of activity and passivity in the anal phase. The phallic phase, which according to Freud occurs between the ages of three and five years, describes how the infant focuses upon its genitals as a source of excitation. It is during the phallic phase that the Oedipus and castration complexes reach their height.

However, it is clear from Freud's *On the Sexual Theories of Children* (1908) that his discussions of the body and its relations to psychical development remain within masculine parameters (1908: 215). Freud postulates that for both sexes during the phallic phase, the genital is perceived as the penis. Furthermore, the infant in its focus upon its genitals considers itself, its mother and all others to possess a penis. For the infant, passage through the phallic phase is brought about by a fear of castration, which, according to Freud, serves to create marked differences between girls and boys in terms of their resultant psychic structures. I will discuss this below in the section on the Oedipus complex.

Freud emphasised, in his discussion of infantile sexuality and development, the different body parts, namely the oral, anal and phallic zones. He described that the development of neurosis occurs when the biologically given libido regresses and becomes fixated to these bodily parts. In his essay, 'Neurosis and Psychosis' (1924), Freud described how the ego is reluctant to accept the powerful force of the id and further defends itself against instinctual impulses by the mechanism of repression. The repressed material creates, as Freud states, a 'substitutive representation' (1924a: 150) in the form of a symptom. The instinctual impulse, or the libido, must withdraw from the ego and needs to find some way of discharging its cathexis of energy. Freud states in 'The Paths to the Formation of Symptoms' (1917), how the libido must withdraw from the ego. It then regresses by forming a fixation on its route of earlier development. These activities and experiences constitute the oral, anal and phallic stages of development. Through the process of fixation to these bodily parts, the libido finds satisfaction.

## Pleasure and unpleasure

Freud's discussions of the body and its correlation with psychical processes feature in his theories of mental processes and ego-formation. Freud's first account of mental processes was in his unpublished *Project for a Scientific*

*Psychology* (1895). His first published account of mental processes appears in *The Interpretation of Dreams* in 1900. In this text, Freud discusses the unconscious and its dominance by pleasure principle. Mental functioning for Freud consists of two mechanisms in which the body is involved. First, is the avoidance of pain whereby unpleasant tension is discharged. Second, is the aim towards pleasure, which occurs, as a result of the discharging of unpleasure. Elizabeth Wright states that, in Freudian theory, bodily needs are connected to the feelings of pleasure and pain which, in turn, affect the mind: 'The mind comes into being out of the body. What is necessarily given at the start is the needs of the body itself: these are inseparably connected to feelings of pleasure and pain' (Wright 1984: 10).

When the body interacts and experiences the external reality of the outside world, the part of the mind Freud names as the ego, then serves to represent the needs of the body. The ego refers to the instinct of self-preservation. The individual has to comply with the demands of the external social world. Therefore, the ego has to control the 'id', which represents the pleasure seeking sexual instinct or libidinal drive within the body. Wright states, 'this is viewed as a struggle between the 'reality principle' and the 'pleasure principle', in which the body has to learn to postpone pleasure and accept a degree of unpleasure in order to comply with social demands' (ibid.).

## Ego-formation and the body

Freud offers two versions of the ego: the narcissistic ego and the realist ego. These versions of the ego appear intermittently through his work. In *Three Essays on the Theory of Sexuality* (1905b), Freud expresses the necessity to explain the genesis of the ego, which he offers later in *On Narcissism: An Introduction* in 1914. Freud states that the formation of the ego begins, for the infant, in the realm of narcissism. Up until the infant is about six months old, it perceives its body as a continuum of the mother or primary carer; it has no sense of being distinct. Freud specifies that in this narcissistic stage, the libidinal impulses in the infant's body are free flowing and uncontained. The infant retains its libido within its own body and has the ability to take itself, or part of its own body, as a libidinal, or rather, love object. Freud refers to this as the ego-libido. The ego, containing libidinal energies, also finds external objects in which to invest them, which Freud refers to as the 'object-libido'.

In *The Ego and the Id*, Freud confirms his statements made in *On Narcissism*. He describes the ego at this stage as predominately a body-ego: 'The ego is first and foremost a bodily ego; it is not merely a surface entity, but is itself the projection of a surface' (1923: 26). The ego is formed, or is a result of, internal libidinal bodily sensations and intensities experienced by the infant. Grosz usefully refers to the ego as representing a kind of 'bodily tracing' or 'psychical map of the body's libidinal intensities' (Grosz 1994: 33). Freud's theory of the narcissistic beginnings of the ego suggests that a person can never be indifferent to their bodies. The body is not something that is merely functional, rather, the body 'must maintain a certain level of psychical and libidinal investment' (ibid.: 32).

The infant then begins to have a sense of the external world beyond its own body. It can begin to distinguish between its insides and the external world beyond its own skin boundaries. As Grosz states, the sexual drives start to emerge and begin to 'distinguish themselves in their specificity, first according to the particular sites or erotogenic zones of the body (oral, anal, phallic, scopophilic, etc.) from which they emanate; and then with particular sources, aims and objects' (Grosz in Price and Shildrick 1999: 268). External objects now represent a status for the infant outside of its own body. The infant can now gain a sense of its own identity. The infant's ego is determined through its relations with others, particularly its primary carer. The infant will strive to identify with others and introject these images into its ego in the form of the ego ideal. Therefore, Freud specifies that the ego and its formation, lies in a position between innate bodily processes and the social world.

Freud's concept of the realist ego appears in *The Interpretation of Dreams* in 1900 and in *The Ego and The Id* in 1923. The realist ego relates to that which intervenes between the erratic, passionate id, and external reality: 'The ego represents what may be called reason and common sense, in contrast to the id, which contains the passions' (1923: 25). The id, according to Freud, is an expression of the biological instincts and is also unconscious.

Freud suggests that the relation between the ego and the id reflects the image of a rider of a horse. The horse symbolises the id, which needs to be kept under control by the rider. The primary role of the realist ego is to control the unreasonable demands of the id and to protect the id from potentially harmful external stimuli. Thus the body contains a continuing negotiation between pleasure, and unpleasure that is imposed by the external world. Consequently, Freud's notion of the development of the ego suggests that the ego represents the infant's relationship and conception of, its own body, the outside world, and other people. This reveals that psychoanalytic theory is not just concerned with the 'inner' psychical processes. As Freud's notion of the development of the ego shows, it is also concerned with the outside social world, and the body is positioned as a mediator between the two.

## The Oedipus complex

Freud identifies the primary love object of the little boy as his mother. According to the boy, his mother's body is phallic. She is in possession of a penis. The boy experiences feelings of rivalry with his father for her affections. Accordingly, the function of the Oedipus complex for the boy is to repress his desire for the mother, and to eventually identify with his father, thus taking up a masculine position in the world. Freud formulated his theory of the Oedipus complex through a process of self-analysis, and in a letter to his friend Fliess he wrote of his feelings of jealously towards his father and being in love with his mother.

During the phallic phase, the boy's preoccupation with his penis and masturbatory activities are regularly met with disapproval from adults. However, according to Freud, the boy is proud of his penis and therefore fails to fully respond to his parents' anxieties. It is only when he observes that the females around him do not possess a penis that his anxieties begin. According to Freud, the boy assumes that the females he encounters in the world have been castrated and were once in possession of a penis. Consequently, the boy fears that his father will castrate him. Upon seeing the absence of a penis in his mother or sister, for example, the boy imagines that they have been castrated by the father and fears the same will happen to him. This entry into the castration complex marks for Freud the conclusion of the Oedipus complex for the boy. The boy is forced to give up his desire for his mother through his fears of castration. Consequently, he represses his Oedipal love for his mother and forms identification with his previously threatening father, which he in turn internalises and, according to Freud, this marks the formation of the boy's super-ego.

## Freud and femininity: the body as masculine

The girl, according to Freud, also experiences her phallic mother as her primary love object but has to give up this desire in order to take the position of 'normal' femininity. Freud states that the girl has to pass through a succession of stages to reach a feminine position. One of these stages is characterised by the girl having to give up her clitoris, from which she derives pleasure, which Freud considers as masculine. Freud states that upon comparing herself to the boy, the girl sees her clitoris as a small penis. Freud describes the young girl, in his essay 'Femininity', as 'a little man' (1933: 118) whose masturbatory activity is focused upon what is described by Freud as a 'penis-equivalent' (ibid.). Thus the girl's body, from the beginning, is perceived as being within a masculine, and inferior masculine position. The girl, according to Freud, has to replace her masculine clitoris with her feminine vagina, which thus becomes her leading genital zone.

According to Freud, the castration complex for the girl constitutes her entry into the Oedipus complex. Upon recognising the anatomical difference between herself and boys and, seeing the penis as a universal organ, the girl feels deprived by her lack of a penis. Freud suggests in *Some Psychical Consequences of the Anatomical Distinction Between the Sexes*

(1925), that the girl understands her lack of a penis by assuming she once possessed a penis (in equal size to the boy's penis) but had lost it by castration. The girl who has previously been both psychically and physically attached to her mother starts to blame her mother for her lack.

According to Freud, the girl turns to her father in the hope of gaining possession of a penis and consequently develops a feeling of envy towards the men around her for their possession of a penis. Freud states that in conjunction with her feelings of penis envy the girl abandons her clitoral masturbation. She realises, according to Freud, that she cannot compete with boys and feels humiliated by her lack: 'the little girl's recognition of the anatomical distinction between the sexes forces her away from masculinity and masculine masturbation on to new lines which lead to the development of femininity' (1925: 256). The girl perceives her father as her love object and experiences hostility and jealousy towards her mother. Freud suggests that the girl's desire for a penis translates into a wish to bear her father's child. If the child is a boy then this, according to Freud, is an ultimate fulfilment for a woman, as the male child brings with him the longed-for penis.

Freud states that females remain in the Oedipus complex for an unspecified length of time and may never completely abandon it. For the boy, the fear of castration by his father initiates him into leaving the Oedipal stage, but for the girl this motive is absent. She experiences her castration anxiety prior to the Oedipus stage and, according to Freud, 'enters the Oedipus situation as though into a haven of refuge' (1933: 129).

## Freud and women's mental distress as penis envy

Freud considers that the Oedipus complex for both sexes is vital for personality development and sexual orientation. The girl, for instance, has to replace her mother as love object, with her father in order to take up the position of 'normal' femininity and a heterosexual position. In addition, the girl has to successfully pass through this stage to avoid neurosis and other mental distress. Freud stresses that there are three possible courses following the girl's realisation of her castration. First, she can take up a normal feminine position by passing successfully through the Oedipus complex. Second, she may develop neurosis or sexual inhibition as a result of repressing her unconscious desire for a penis, which, according to Freud, 'persists in the unconscious and retains a considerable amount of energy. The wish to get the longed-for penis eventually in spite of everything may contribute to the motives that drive a mature woman to analysis' (1933: 125). Third, according to Freud, the girl may develop a 'masculinity complex' whereby she regresses back to her early masculinity stage, when her leading genital zone was her clitoris, through her incapacity to accept her castration and lack of a penis.

During the three stages of psychosexual development, the body, for Freud, is a zone of excitation or an auto-erotic zone. As with the hysterical body, the infant's body is a site of sexual pleasure. In his discussions of the genital phase, Freud positions the body in male parameters. The female has to abandon her masculine zone of pleasure and has to opt for the feminine vagina to become normal. Thus, for Freud, psychical health depends on which part of her body the girl chooses for sexual pleasure. Furthermore, even if the female does adopt the normal feminine position, she remains as lacking. For Freud, a repressed longing for a penis can have severe consequences for a woman's psychical life. These theories have been criticised by feminist thinkers who consider them to be biologically determinist.

## Biological determinism: feminism's attack on Freud

Because of his theory of the Oedipus complex and his contention that women perceive their bodies as inferior due to their lack of a penis, Freud has come under attack from various thinkers including the second wave feminists of the 1970s. In the US, feminists including Betty Friedan, Shulamith Firestone and Kate Millett condemned Freud and his theories on femininity. The American psychiatric establishments were, at that time, highly influenced by Freudian thought and the ground for opposing such theories was set in the climate of political and social movements such as those concerning Civil Rights, the New Left and anti-psychiatry. The arguments against Freudian thought staged by Friedan, Firestone and Millett were concerned with the ways in which female subordination was perceived to have little to do with biology, but was, rather, the result of social construction. Kate Millett, for example, in her book *Sexual Politics*, which was published in 1970, argued that female subordination is internalised from ideological structures within social institutions such as the family.

Millett criticises Freud for basing his theories of women on his universal concept of penis envy. Millett accepts that Freud's patients were likely to have expressed feelings of inferiority as he describes, but he fails to acknowledge the social and economic disadvantages of women that may cause such feelings. According to Millett, Freud focuses on purely biological explanations and considers the young girl's discovery that she is lacking a penis, and her subsequent feelings of castration, as a major catastrophe that will have a profound effect upon her future psychical development. Millett states that Freud's seemingly limited focus upon the biological has influenced subsequent psychological and psychoanalytic thought: 'His entire psychology of women, from which all modern psychology and psychoanalysis derives heavily, is built upon an original tragic experience-born female' (1970: 180).

Millett argues that Freud's theory of the castration experience of girls is a synthesis of unexplained assumptions. For instance, Millett asks why the girl automatically sees her smaller clitoris as inferior and the boy's penis as superior: 'Why is the girl instantly struck by the proposition that bigger is better?' (ibid.: 181). Millett argues that it would be equally feasible that the girl may view her own body as the norm as the boy so obviously does in Freud's consideration. Additionally, Millett argues that young children must initially perceive the mother's body and her breasts, which are absent in the father's body. Millett considers that this anatomical fact is overlooked in Freudian theory with his focus upon the apparent importance of the possession of a penis for both sexes. Millett puts forward further criticism and points out that according to Freud, the girl blames her mother for her lack of penis, gives up hope of impregnating her and subsequently turns to her father. Millett questions how young children can possess such awareness of conception, which she contends is a complex process that not all adults can successfully work out.

Freud's discussions of the way in which bearing a son can bring a woman fulfilment of the longed-for penis, is considered by Millett as disparaging towards a woman's capacity to bear children. Stating that the accomplishment of childbirth should be praised, Millett argues that Freud reduces it 'into nothing more than a hunt for the male organ' (ibid.: 185). Millett states that these theories are used to justify the subservient position of women in relation to men whereby a woman's genetic identity is her destiny. Millett argues that Freud dismissed the opportunity to examine the consequences of patriarchal culture upon the evolving female ego, but instead chose to justify female oppression with biological explanations.

What Millett does not discuss in detail are Freud's early accounts of his female patients suffering from hysteria. She alludes to them and states that through his clinical work with women, 'Freud did not accept his patients' symptoms as evidence of a justified dissatisfaction with the limiting circumstances imposed upon them by society' (ibid.: 179). Millett suggests that, instead, Freud explained women's symptoms as due to penis envy. Yet, as I have suggested, Freud presents these early female patients as subjects and suggests that conflicts between their sexual desire and ties to domesticity, imposed upon them by their families and so forth, are manifested in their bodies. He thus goes beyond biological explanations in explaining their distress. These accounts also appeared over a decade before Freud's first mention of penis envy in *On the Sexual Theories of Children* in 1908 (Laplanche and Pontalis 1988: 30).

## Conclusion

Freud's writings emphasise the body and its relationship with psychical processes. In his early writings, and in a radical shift away from preceding accounts of the aetiology of hysteria, Freud suggests that hysteria represents a translation of repressed, psychical conflict that cannot be communicated by verbal means. The accounts of hysterical symptoms preceding Freud, considered the female body as dangerous and uncontrollable. Freud suggested that such symptoms are valuable and meaningful to the lived experiences of women. He suggested that women experience conflict between their ties to the domestic sphere and their desires, and Freud showed how these conflicts are manifested in their bodies. He appeared to remain dedicated to his notion that symptoms have a specific meaning relating to the lived experience of the individual presenting them.

Freud's notion of the ego as initially a bodily ego indicates that our sense of self emerges from our early experiences of our bodily sensations through which we learn about what is inside and outside. Subsequently, through contact with our primary carer and the outside world, we form our own identity and autonomy. These processes are also essential to the development and current experience of a person's sense of self. Freud's writings on infantile sexuality argue that the body is a site of innumerable erotogenic zones through which the infant develops psychically, establishes its identity, and learns to relate to the external world. Neurosis is an effect of the biologically given libido being fixated to oral, anal or genital body parts. Freud's theories on the Oedipus complex and femininity however, position the female body within masculine parameters. Freud represents the needs of the female body, in his writings on femininity and penis envy, as being psychically and physically motivated towards acquiring the male genital organ. Consequently, Freud considers women's mental distress as being largely due to envy of the penis.

As I have stated, rather than merely stemming from a specific mental illness with a meaningless biological cause, Freud argues that symptoms are significant and have symbolic meaning for the lived experiences of the individual. In working with people who experience mental illness, we might consider that they may have painful experiences that are too distressing to put into words. Many people, understandably, do not want to talk about certain experiences, especially if they are painful. However, in the understanding of patients we might want to pay attention to their bodily expressions that might communicate something to us about them. In understanding our patients, we might work with them in a more informed and therapeutic way (I discuss this in more detail in Chapter 9). Importantly, we can make sense of their mental distress in the context of their lives, rather than merely attributing biological explanations, which of course have a valuable place. In the case of 'neurosis', then, painful or distressing thoughts are repressed, or as I suggested earlier, swallowed down and then emerge in the form of a 'symptom' that is often bodily. In the case of psychosis, the experience, which often has not yet become a thought, is expelled and emerges as if from outside and is perceived in a concrete manner. In the next chapter, I will discuss post-Freudian accounts of the body in psychosis.

# Chapter 6

# Psychosis

In the last chapter, I outlined the work of Freud and his emphasis upon the correlations between psychical and physical processes. The body is presented by Freud as a container for repressed psychical conflicts and therefore as a site for the non-verbal communication of these. Freud also focuses upon the body in his account of the development of the ego. As I hope I have shown, Freud's notions of the body are relevant because he places importance on symptoms as relating to the lived experience of the individual rather than to an organic cause. In his understanding of 'neurotic' conditions including hysteria (now commonly referred to as conversion), depression, anxiety and so on, the distressing experience is swallowed down or taken inside and seemingly hidden, only to be revealed in a symptom. This symptom – often expressed bodily, as we have seen – is created by the person as a way to help them, to put it simply, bear being alive.

In this chapter I will discuss the body in psychosis, outlining the work of a variety of post-Freudian theorists. I will demonstrate how they apply their concepts to an understanding of the bodily experiences of people with psychosis. As I stated in the introduction, in my practice I have observed in the patients we call 'psychotic' or 'schizophrenic', a particular way of being. Often there is a blurring between inside and outside, and there is a feeling that outside people or things are merging with them, or that they are merging with things or other people outside. To me, some of the photographs by Francesca Woodman (1958–1981) seem to depict this experience. They show her blurred body being merged and disappearing into fragmented buildings.

Very commonly in psychosis, there is a feeling of being invaded, spied upon, controlled or attacked from outside. We do indeed know that brain chemical imbalance can produce psychotic symptoms. However, it is also interesting to look at the relationship between someone's life experiences and their symptoms. The perspectives outlined in this chapter, although often tiresome and long-winded, suggest that psychotic symptoms relate to factors primarily stemming from experiences of early life, or in Laing's estimation, of simply being alive. I hope they provoke the mental health practitioner to look beyond diagnosis and consider the life experiences of patients, and ways in which these experiences sometimes cause people to relate to the world in a certain (seemingly strange and curious) way.

## Schilder and body image

Paul Schilder's work during the 1920s and 1930s on body image is largely influenced by psychoanalysis. For Schilder, body image is a construct made up of libidinal and psychical representations. It is influenced by the amount of libidinal energy the individual has invested in his or her body, as well as by social and emotional factors. Like Freud, Schilder discusses how the infant's first object of primary narcissism is the image of the body. The infant projects bodily sensations onto the outside world and intro-jects the external world into its body. Schilder discusses the stages of infan-tile development outlined by Freud involving the oral, anal and genital body parts. Each stage involves an investment of libidinal energy and thus influences the formation of the body image: 'There will be lines of energy connecting the different erotogenic points, and we shall have a variation in the structure of the body-image according to the psychosexual tendencies of the individual' (Schilder 1978: 126).

Like Freud, Schilder states that an individual's body image is formed by the physical sensations it experiences. At first, the infant's body image is confused with others and it then forms an identity of its own. The forma-tion of the body image is also influenced by the hopes and fears the primary carer projects into the infant's body. The infant will internalise these during its early development. The mother or primary carer will invest certain feelings into the body of her infant and, following this, the infant's body image will undergo certain modifications during the course of its development.

The body image, according to Schilder, can greatly alter with the onset of psychological or physical pain. An individual with hypochondria for example, will overly invest a certain region of their body with libidinal energy. This particular body part will take on the status of a genital zone. The hypochondriac attempts to reject the libidinally invested body part so that it is not included within the individual's complete body image: 'the individual defends himself against the libidinous overtension of the hypochondriac organ; he tries to isolate the diseased organ, to treat it like a foreign body in the body-image' (ibid.: 142).

Schilder describes the condition of depersonalisation as consisting of a lack of interest in the whole body. This can be an early symptom of schizophrenia whereby the outside world is experienced as unreal. The individual's thinking and sense of self are experienced as mechanical. Unlike the hypochondriac, the individual experiencing depersonalisation will exhibit a refusal to invest any libidinal energy into their body, leading to alterations in their conception of themselves and of the external world. These individuals will not feel centred within their bodies and may view themselves as if from outside. In psychotic depersonalisation, individuals experience their bodies as being controlled, invaded or infested by external agencies. Psychotic people will often experience delusions that their body parts are controlled by an outside force, or may believe that an animal inhabits their body, or that an outside force is invading them. Schilder further discusses his concept of the body image in his book, *On Psychoses* (1976) to which I will now turn.

The defence mechanism of projection serves to construct a person's perception and experience of the world around them. In early life, according to Schilder, the infant's sense of its own body does not always correspond with its perception of the outside world. When the infant experiences something, it may not know which parts belong to its own body, or to the outside world. The infant's tendency to project onto the outside world is necessary for the formation of its identity. Some bodily parts or excretions, such as saliva and milk, retain some relation to the infant's body, but the process of expelling the faeces tends to blend with the process of projection.

Schilder takes up Freud's concept of the psychotic individual who withdraws libido from outside objects and invests it in their own body as a narcissistic ego. The psychotic person will also undergo a process of excessive introjection whereby outside objects are taken in as part of an individual's personality or body. Movements and experiences in the outer world can also be perceived as part of their body. Clothes or implements are often perceived to be part of one's body. In usual circumstances, outside objects become part of the body image, such as a driver in a car. Within schizoid states of mind this is more exaggerated. Schilder describes a patient who specified how she observed somebody sweeping the street and experienced it as a sweeping of her genitals. Another patient thought that his penis was lying on the street and crushed by cars or taken away by dogs. These experiences can signify that outer objects are being introjected into the individual's body, and can also suggest that the individual has projected a part of their body as an outside object, which is experienced as damaged by outside forces (Schilder 1976: 22).

In depersonalisation, individuals lose interest in their bodies, as there is reluctance for narcissistic investment in the body. Love of the body, as the individual lives it, enables the preservation and maintenance of the body in the carrying out of actions such as washing and dressing. A particular so-called 'negative symptom' of schizophrenia is self-neglect whereby the patient does not appear interested in attending to hygiene and self-care. From a psychoanalytic perspective, one can say that these individuals have no libidinal investment in their bodies. With this in mind, it would be useless to say to a patient: 'Go and have a wash, you'll feel better!' The clinician could not expect the patient to suddenly feel interested in their body in response to such a remark. They might work differently with the patient by understanding this lack of sense of being in, or owning the body, and consequently being reluctant to care for his or her body.

## Lacan: body as real, imaginary and symbolic

I will now outline Jacques Lacan's writings about the body – as real, imaginary and symbolic. I will also give an account of various applications of these concepts to the understanding of the structure of psychosis. I will begin with Lacan's concept of ego formation in the mirror stage and his outline of the Oedipus complex.

### The pre-Oedipal stage

Upon separation from our mother, or primary carer, we acquire a sense of what is inside of us and what is outside of us. For the first six months of life, according to Lacan, the infant experiences oneness with its mother's body and has no concept of its own ego boundaries. This stage is termed by Lacan as the pre-Oedipal stage. Lacan, like Freud, states that during this stage libidinal energies (which are perhaps something like a life instinct or life force) circulate around the infant's body.

The mother or the maternal figure meets the infant's biological needs. However, according to Lacan, the pre-Oedipal relationship does not just consist of an infant and mother dyad. There is, in addition, always a third party, namely the imaginary phallus that the mother desires. In his seminar of 1957–1958, Lacan refers to this three-way relationship as the 'first' time of the Oedipus complex. I shall return to this in my discussion of the Oedipus complex below, with an attempt to provide a definition of Lacan's phallus as not referring to a biological penis. I will now turn to Lacan's concept of the mirror stage.

### The mirror stage

According to Lacan, the ego (or sense of self) begins to emerge at the mirror stage when the infant is about six months old. At this stage, the infant begins to experience itself as distinct from its mother and experiences a lack of her presence, which is of course the infant's first experience of separation. Due to this perceived absence, the infant's biological needs and demands are, as Grosz describes, 'converted into social, imaginary, and linguistic forms' (Grosz 1990: 60). In other words, the infant's early relationships take many forms. The relationship is based on the 'real' presence of the parents, and the infant's perceptions of them that are often imaginary. Also, as we shall see, in Lacan's estimation, language is an essential component of this early relationship. When the infant begins to separate from the mother, it directs its needs and demands onto her as a separate being. This is necessary because it ensures a process whereby the infant becomes a separate subject, and is able to perceive others.

Two processes mark the formation of the infant's ego. First, individuals with whom the infant forms its identity, such as the mother's body or the infant's own reflection of itself in the mirror, are introjected (or in other words, taken inside) onto the ego as an 'ego ideal'. Second, the libidinal energies previously circulating in the infant's body are blocked or redirected. This enables the infant to form a narcissistic attachment to its body or part of itself. This is, of course, necessary to being a separate being in the world. It is not just about self-love; it is also about valuing oneself in relation to others. Grosz states that this process enables subjects to form and maintain a relation of love (or hate) towards their bodies: 'The body is libidinally invested ... Its value is never simply or solely functional, for it has a (libidinal) value in itself' (1994: 32).

Similarly to Freud, Lacan proposes that the ego is formed from the body. The ego comes into being as a projection of the infant's perceived bodily experience in relations to others, from its internal and external perception of itself. However, he proposes that the infant perceives its body not as it really is. The infant perceives it in terms of what Lacan refers to as its imaginary anatomy. At the mirror stage, the infant, when encountering its reflection in the mirror, sees its body as complete and unified. This image is preserved after the Oedipus complex. This is the ego ideal to which the ego will always strive as this unified body suggests a stable and unified ego. According to Lacan, the infant, upon observing its unified mirror image, experiences jubilation and a sense of bodily mastery. However, according to Lacan, this is imagined and a misconception as it is not synonymous with the infant's real bodily experiences. The infant is, in fact, developmentally immature with regards to coordination and gaining control over its bodily processes. The infant therefore experiences its body as fragmented, as what Lacan refers to as the 'body-in-bits-and-pieces'.

The infant's real experience of its body as fragmented engenders friction and aggression towards its unified image in the mirror. In order to resolve this tension, the infant identifies with the unified image. This identification brings about joy initially for the infant, but there may follow a depressive response when it compares its own achievements with its omnipotent mother as desiring the phallus. The infant will however strive to identify with the unified other. This will give the infant a sense of its own (albeit imaginary) unified, fixed sense of self, as Grosz states: 'The ego illusory sees itself as autonomous and self-determined, independent of otherness. It feels itself to be its own origin, unified and developed *in/by nature*' (1990: 43). The infant's perception of itself as a distinct subject enables to its entry into the symbolic order to which I will now turn.

## The symbolic order and the name-of-the-father

The Lacanian concept of the infant's entry into the symbolic order (which refers to the realm of language and subjectivity) constitutes Freud's Oedipus complex rewritten to include a linguistic emphasis. One major difference between Freud and Lacan concerns the penis. Freud focuses upon the penis as a biological organ that the young girl envies and desires. Lacan adopts the term 'phallus' to describe, as Dylan Evans points out, the role the biological penis plays in fantasy. The phallus therefore represents 'the imaginary and symbolic functions' (Evans 1996: 140) of the biological penis. The phallus is described by Lacan to be representative of language and a signifier of desire. He explains this in his essay, 'The Signification of the Phallus' (1977: 285). The phallus is the essential signifier in relation to which the infant attains its identity as a speaking 'I'. The individual is placed in relation to the phallus by what Lacan terms as the name-of-the-father.

As I have discussed, Lacan describes the first six months of the child's life as the pre-Oedipal stage whereby the infant experiences itself as continuous with its mother's body. However, Lacan does not see this stage as a relation between two people. Rather, it also involves a third party, which he describes as the presence of the imaginary phallus. The mother is, in fact, a 'phallic' mother, so termed as she carries an unconscious desire for the phallus she lacks. In the Oedipal stage, according to Lacan, the phallus comes to be perceived by the infant as the primary object of desire in the mother, beyond the infant. Consequently, the infant attempts to identify with the imaginary phallus in order to satisfy its mother's desire and to fill her lack, as stated by Lacan: 'If the desire of the mother *is* the phallus, then the child wishes to be the phallus so to satisfy this desire' (Lacan in Mitchell and Rose 1982: 83).

The phallic object of the mother's desire is perceived by the infant as omnipotent. However, at this stage both the mother and infant are marked by lack. The mother lacks the desired phallus, and the infant, who seeks to be the phallus to satisfy her, recognises that realisation of this desire is impossible. The child consequently wishes to present something to its mother in the real but recognises its own biological organ (male or female) to be inadequate. Recognition of impotence and inadequacy brings about anxiety in the infant, who is also faced by the threat of the omnipotent object of its mother's desire. This stage is followed by the intervention of the imaginary father.

Lacan proposes that the father is perceived by the infant as imaginary in the second 'time' of the Oedipus stage. By imposing the law, the imaginary father denies the mother the desired phallus (and thereby symbolically castrates her), and denies the infant access to the mother. Through language, the mother relates to the infant her satisfaction with the father's intervention. Thus, the infant is faced with the father as rival for the mother's desire.

In the third 'time' of the Oedipus scenario the real father emerges and reveals he has the phallus. The real father prevents the infant from further attempting to be the phallus in order to satisfy the mother's desire. He thus provokes and reinforces the incest taboo, and thereby symbolically castrates the infant. The infant is freed from the anxiety of trying to be the phallus. He sees the father as possessing it, identifies with the father, and accepts his mother's lack of a phallus. Upon separating from the mother, the infant has no further wish to satisfy her lack. The infant identifies with the-name-of-the-father who positions it as a speaking 'I' within the symbolic order that constitutes the realm of subjectivity and language.

Charles W. Bonner points out that the body continues to be significant in Lacan's concept of the symbolic, just as it is in his concept of the mirror stage. The infant's emerging imaginary sense of its body and self as unified is considered by Lacan as a defence against the anxiety of its real fragmented experience. In the Oedipal stage when the infant enters the symbolic these fragmented body images serve to bring about castration anxiety in the infant. According to Bonner, Lacanian theory states how the infant, through language, names its different body parts and having or not having the penis is of particular concern (Bonner in Welton 1999: 244). Fear of bodily harm or fragmentation becomes apparent in castration anxiety to which I will now turn.

Like Freud, Lacan considers the Oedipus complex to produce opposing psychic characteristics for boys and girls. Lacan states that to enter into the symbolic order, both sexes are required to abandon desire for the mother as primary love object. The mother's castration must be accepted and the infant must acquire a speaking position separately from the mother's body. The infant can only acquire and maintain this position with reference to the law, or the name-of-the-father. As Lacan states: 'It is the *name-of-the-father* that we may recognise as the support of the symbolic function, which, from the dawn of history has identified his person with the figure of the law' (1977: 67). The infant is thus positioned within the symbolic order by introjecting the father's name and by becoming a speaking 'I'.

It appears that this process is more straightforward for the male infant. According to Lacan, the girl is in a position of being castrated like her mother. This means that she has a passive role within the symbolic order, and her subjectivity is more precarious. Lacan asserts that as the phallus signifies desire, the female is positioned in relation to the signifier, which places her in a position of 'being' the phallus rather than 'having' it. The girl then becomes an object of desire for the male subject. Lacan states that women must necessarily appear to be the phallus in order for men to be seen as having it. Lacan considers that women appear to be the phallus through masquerade, imitation and mimesis. They thereby imitate the male subject.

## Psychosis and ego-formation

Lacan's outline of ego-formation and the Oedipus complex reveal correlations between psychical and physical processes. I will now discuss how Lacan and other theorists have applied these concepts to the understanding of psychosis. The formation of the ego, necessary in order for the infant to perceive itself as a distinct and unified subject, is created from the infant's perception of its own body. The infant identifies with its imagined unified image but in reality it experiences its body as fragmented. Lacan asserts that remnants of these real experiences are often present in the dreams of so-called 'normal' individuals. Such dreams, Lacan argues, are of a body in disarray like those depicted in the paintings of Hieronymus Bosch that portray disjointed and uncoordinated bodies.

Lacan suggests that such images are present in the symptoms of psychosis. In psychotic states of mind people experience themselves, and consequently their bodies, in fragments, which they often experience as outside of themselves and as threatening. In Lacanian terms, the psychotic individual is positioned in the pre-imaginary real. The sense of self, or the ego, is not unified which would normally occur as a result of identification with the unified mirror image. The individual rather experiences its sense of self in the real, in relation to the stage whereby the infant experiences its body as fragmented.

## Caillois on space

In his essay, 'The Mirror Stage as Formative of the Function of the I' (in Lacan 1977), Lacan refers to the work of Roger Caillois who discusses the position of the individual in relation to space in an essay entitled, 'Mimicry and Legendary Psychasthenia'. Caillois states that complete occupation in the space taken up by the body is vital for an individual to become, and experience himself or herself as, a subject. He suggests that for the psychotic, the situation of experiencing the self in the body, and the space the body inhabits, is problematic: 'To these dispossessed souls, space seems to be a devouring force ... Then the body separates itself from thought, the individual breaks the boundary of his skin and occupies the other side of his senses' (Caillois in Grosz 1994: 47).

The psychotic person, therefore, does not feel located in the right place. The sense of self is fragmented causing them to observe themselves from the outside of their bodies, or to hear the voices of others and to experience alienation from outside forces. One can therefore identify themes in Caillois' work that appear to have influenced Lacan and his concept of the mirror stage. The ability to locate oneself in an affirmative space marks the success of the resolution of the mirror stage, as Grosz states: 'Only through the resolution of the mirror-stage dilemmas of identity, when the child becomes able to distinguish itself definitively from objects and above all from others, can this space be attained' (1994: 48). From my own clinical work and observations, it is clear that some people with psychosis do experience their bodies, or rather their subjectivity, in these ways. Experiences of being controlled by outside forces or hearing another's voice either inside or outside one's head seems to suggest that the ego is somehow not unified.

## Bowie and foreclosure

With regard to the Oedipus complex and psychosis, Lacan proposes that psychosis occurs when the individual forecloses the 'parental metaphor' or the-name-of-the-father in the symbolic. Malcolm Bowie states that foreclosure is indicative of a psychotic state whereby there is a getting rid of something in the unconscious. This is in contrast to repression which is related to neurosis: 'Where foreclosure seeks to expel a given notion, thought, image, memory or signifier from the unconscious, repression seeks to confine it there' (Bowie 1991: 107).

According to Lacan, the name-of-the-father having been foreclosed stands in symbolic opposition to the individual. That which is foreclosed returns in the real in the form of hallucinations and delusions. Psychosis occurs when the individual attempts to fill the gap, usually filled by the missing name-of-the-father, in the symbolic realm:

> It is the lack of the Name-of-the-Father in that place which, by the hole that it opens up in the signified, sets off the cascade of reshapings of the signifier from which the increasing disaster of the imaginary proceeds, to the point at which the level is reached at which signifier and signified are stabilized in the delusional metaphor.
>
> (Lacan 1977: 217)

The phallus may feature in psychotic thinking whereby it is not felt to be part of the individual's self or body but is projected out and experienced as an external threatening force. In addition, the psychotic person, in Lacanian terms, is positioned within a pre-verbal realm, whereby they have not identified with or introjected the name-of-the-father and consequently have not been positioned as a speaking 'I'. Therefore, the mirror stage has not been negotiated and passed through. The body is experienced in bits and pieces and this also marks the stage whereby the infant is still trying to be the phallus to satisfy its mother's lack, rather than identifying with it.

## Concluding Lacan

Lacan's (challenging) writings on the body reveal ways in which the body has meaning for the individual. A sense of self comes into being from the individual's internal and external perceptions. Lacan's outline of the mirror stage indicates that a unified, stable ego or sense of self is fragile for most of us and has to be reinforced and affirmed by our relations to others. For the psychotic individual, the sense of self as a complete and secure unity has never occurred. Parts of the self are felt to be on the outside and are often threatening and invasive. For Lacan, these symbolise the name-of-the-father in opposition, who normally stands to position the infant in the realm of subjectivity and as a distinct, speaking 'I'. These ideas on the structure of psychosis, take into account the lived experiences of an individual. Lacan pointed out in his doctoral dissertation on paranoia written in 1932, that psychiatric practice shows a disregard for the subject's experience and speech. He states that the term paranoia is meaningless unless understood in relation to the subject's personality. Similarly to Freud, Lacan's writings on the body and mental distress appear to attach meanings to symptoms that specifically relate to the individual's life and experience. In contrast, as I pointed out in Chapter 3, psychiatry tends to focus upon symptoms as determined by biology rather than as psychologically meaningful, not least in terms of the body, its experience and representation.

## French feminism

Two theorists, Luce Irigaray and Julia Kristeva, often referred to as 'French feminists' or 'psychoanalytic feminists', appear to be both influenced by, and critical of, Freudian and particularly, Lacanian psychoanalytic thought. They state that women are considered as the 'other' in relation to the phallus, and the expressions of their sexuality and identity are therefore tenuous. Irigaray and Kristeva further explore women's position in relation to the symbolic, and their emphasis centres on the female body, language and identity.

### Irigaray on woman as the other sex

The work of Irigaray has largely been concerned with the discussion of dominant, patriarchal discourses and the ways in which these have been reproduced historically. Irigaray has coined the term 'sameness' to describe how discourses of, for example, philosophy and psychoanalysis, have claimed to be sex-neutral but have, in fact, been male-centred. Freudian thought has considered the psychic and sexual development of the individual only from the viewpoint of the male. Irigaray states: 'The feminine is always described in terms of deficiency or atrophy, as the other side of the sex that alone holds the monopoly on value: The male sex' (Irigaray in Whitford 1991: 119).

Irigaray's *Speculum of the Other Woman* (1985a) contains a critique of both Freud and Lacan. Its title refers to Lacan's mirror stage whereby the infant is presented with an image of itself, forms its ego, or sense of self, which it then projects onto the outside world. Irigaray argues that it is the male ego that is projected onto the world, which then becomes a mirror whereby the male can see his own reflection universally. Irigaray suggests an alternative to the flat male mirror and considers one that is curvaceous like the female body and will consequently reflect female experience. As Grosz confirms, Irigaray's female mirror 'represents the other woman, not woman as man's other, but another woman, altogether different from man's other' (1990: 173).

Irigaray argues that within Freudian and Lacanian psychoanalytic thought, there is no emphasis upon female bodily pleasure *as female*. Psychoanalytic thought concerning female sexuality reduces the young girl's desire and pleasure to purely masculine parameters. For example, the so-called 'masculine' clitoris is considered by Freud to be the young girl's primary source of erotic pleasure until she replaces this with the 'feminine' vagina. In response, Irigaray argues that the female body contains multiple sites of erotic pleasure that belong to the feminine and do not serve to reinforce the male organ and its perceived primacy. She states that this point has been overlooked within psychoanalytic discourse: 'Why amputate certain parts of the female genitals? . . . Why retain only those that have, or are supposed to have, their guarantor in the male Sex/organ?' (Irigaray 1985a: 29). Irigaray further elaborates this argument in *This Sex Which is Not One* (1985b), in which she considers the multiplicity of female desire situated in several areas of the female body. Therefore, there is not just 'one' area of desire on the female body. The lips of the vulva are an example of a female sex that is not just 'one': 'Woman touches herself all the time . . . for her genitals are formed of two lips in continuous contact. Thus, within herself, she is already two – but not divisible into one(s) – that caress each other' (1985b: 24).

In addition to the lack of reference in psychoanalytic thought to female pleasure, and the young girl being considered as, in Freud's estimation, a 'little man', Irigaray argues that the female is viewed as a mother, never as a woman. The female, in Freud's estimation, proceeds from desiring a penis, which is then replaced with a desire for a child, in particular a male child who can bring the desired-for penis with him. Irigaray states that the young girl blames her lack of a penis on her mother whom she rejects. This, according to Irigaray, causes the girl to devalue both hers and her mother's sex organs. The mother/daughter and distinctly female relation incorporated within the imaginary and pre-Oedipal stages are overlooked within psychoanalytic discourse. Making reference to Freud's notion of woman as a 'dark continent', she considers the unsymbolised status of the mother/daughter relation, which she sees as a threat to the male symbolic order.

Irigaray argues that patriarchal structures, which serve to repress female sexuality and language, bring about women's madness. As women are outside the symbolic order and therefore do not possess a distinct discourse of their own, Irigaray contends that they cannot speak their suffering. Women's suffering, according to Irigaray, is manifested in their bodies. Providing some clinical examples of this in her paper, 'Women's Exile', she suggests that men tend to suffer more frequently from delusions than women (1977: 74). According to Irigaray, this occurs because women are excluded from language. In her paper, 'Women – Mothers, the Silent Substratum', she states: 'You often need something of language, some delusion, to signal that you are living in madness. Women do not in fact suffer much from delusions . . . they suffer in their bodies' (Irigaray in Whitford 1991: 48). The bodies of women therefore represent a 'feminine syntax', best deciphered in the gestures of women's bodies. However, Irigaray states that deciphering such gestures is problematic because they are often paralysed. She suggests that these gestures are most easily 'read' within the laughter of women, and when women suffer, as in the case of mental distress.

According to Irigaray, the ways in which women psychiatric patients suffer in their bodies reflect the behaviour and presentation of the hysteric. As we have seen with Freud's theories, the hysteric's body is a medium through which the sufferer can state what cannot be translated verbally. Irigaray suggests that the female voice, repressed within patriarchal culture, is revealed in the somatic language of the hysteric. She suggests there is 'a revolutionary potential in hysteria . . . even in her paralysis, the hysteric exhibits a potential for gestures and desires' (ibid.: 47). Irigaray, therefore, celebrates the body of the hysteric as a valuable means of expression of the repressed and unspoken. As outlined above, Irigaray considers female sexuality in terms of fluidity and multiplicity. Female sexuality is not just located in one area of the body. It involves the breasts, labia and the vulva. Here she can be seen to celebrate the movement and fluidity of the body. She thus reapplies, in a feminist context, the patriarchal notions of the wandering womb in Greek culture and beyond, and Freud's discussion of the body as a site of innumerable erotogenic zones.

### Kristeva: the maternal body

Kristeva, in her position as literary theorist and semiologist, draws upon Lacan's concepts of the imaginary and symbolic stages. Kristeva refers to the imaginary or pre-Oedipal stage as the 'semiotic'. The semiotic, according to Kristeva, represents the nameless, rhythmical, undirected grouping of drives that flow in and through the infant's body. Kristeva uses the term 'chora' from Plato's *Timaeus* to describe this process.[1]

Like Freud, Kristeva suggests that the realm of the mother's body dominates this stage. In her essay, 'Revolution in Poetic Language', she describes the drives operating within this realm: 'Drives involve pre-Oedipal semiotic functions and energy discharges that connect and orient the body to the mother' (Kristeva in Moi 1986: 95) According to Kristeva, these drives are biological. As Freud describes, they are instinctual energies consisting of oral and anal drives, which are orientated to the maternal body. On the other hand, Kristeva's notion of the drives is also orientated to, and operates between, the psyche and representation. Kelly Oliver describes this process: 'Kristeva takes up Freud's theory of drives as instinctual energies that operate between biology and culture. Drives have their source in organic tissue and aim at psychological satisfaction' (Oliver in Welton 1999: 342).

Within the realm of the semiotic, the infant develops its sense of identity as a subject and the limits and boundaries of its body. The semiotic represents the pre-patriarchal phase. However, although the semiotic is the enveloping realm of the maternal body, according to Kristeva, it also threatens destruction of the subject. The death drive threatens the subject with engulfment and non-existence. Furthermore, this realm is not entirely feminine.

Kristeva proposes, along with Freud and Lacan, that the mother is phallic. As Grosz states, Kristeva's notion of the mother as phallic lacks a potential celebration of the unique experience of maternity: ' "She" is thus the consequence of a *masculine* fantasy of maternity, rather than women's lived experience of maternity' (Grosz 1990: 151). In *Tales of Love* (1987), Kristeva suggests that maternity is something that is represented rather than experienced. Such representations include the phallocentric Christian images of the Virgin Mother. Kristeva asserts that women can never really inhabit, or speak from the maternal realm. As Grosz states, as mothers, women are unable to articulate their femininity or maternity, they are 'locked within a mute, rhythmic, spasmic, potentially hysterical – and thus speechless – body' (ibid.: 163). I will now turn to Kristeva's notion of the symbolic.

Like Lacan, Kristeva defines the infant's entry into the realm of language and subjectivity as the symbolic. The law of the father governs this realm, and the rhythmic, flowing drives associated with the semiotic are repressed. She maintains that through language, there can be an upsurge or return of the repressed semiotic. However, only men possess this capacity as women are too closely bound with the maternal body. Writers including Joyce, Artaud and Mallarmé exhibit the flowing energies of the semiotic in their work: 'enigmatic and feminine, this space underlying the written is rhythmic, unfettered' (Kristeva in Moi 1986: 97). An ability to represent the semiotic in language, then, belongs to men in their firm position within the symbolic as speaking subjects. Kristeva therefore suggests that it is only those in a stable position (men) within the symbolic who can subvert or transgress it. Men, therefore, can represent the feminine semiotic.

Women writers, according to Kristeva, either produce works that represent the family structure – such as romances or autobiographies – or they write from within their bodies using language that cannot be represented:

'In women's writing, language seems to be from a foreign land; it is seen from the point of view of an asymbolic, spastic body ... Estranged from language, women are visionaries, dancers who suffer as they speak' (Kristeva in Grosz 1990: 165).

Transgression to the realm of the semiotic, or the rupturing of the symbolic, according to Kristeva, threatens potential risks, including psychosis. Like Lacan, Kristeva states that psychosis occurs when the infant forecloses or refuses to represent the name-of-the-father. Therefore, the infant cannot be positioned within the symbolic as a speaking subject. Kristeva suggests that the writers she identifies as representing the maternal semiotic, risk psychosis. These writers may 'presume the place of the mother as repressed – unnameable ... they verge on psychosis' (ibid.). Kristeva seems to suggest that it is only men who risk psychosis in their stable positions within the symbolic. Women, in contrast, are bound to the maternal realm of the semiotic. As Kristeva describes it, the semiotic is unnameable and cannot be represented. It constitutes the realm of the body, with its rhythms and movements. Women's suffering is consequently situated within their bodies. It is suffering that cannot be articulated verbally but through bodily means.

### Concluding French feminism

Irigaray and Kristeva both claim that women are situated outside the patriarchal symbolic order. Positioned as the 'other', a woman's speech is represented as Grosz states 'in a hysterical fury, where the body 'speaks' a discourse that cannot be verbalised by her' (1990: 174). Just as maternity is represented within patriarchal images or fantasies, so too is women's suffering. Irigaray and Kristeva's ideas may be applied to mental health practice. Women's suffering has been represented and articulated by patriarchal structures and institutions, although women's actual experience of suffering is, perhaps, unnameable and often cannot be verbalised by them. Women's suffering, according to Irigaray and Kristeva, is articulated non-verbally in the gestures of the body. These ideas may be applied to my observations of women in Chapter 8. I describe how I sense that the suffering of the women patients I observe is somehow 'stuck inside' of them and cannot be verbalised. When these women speak about their bodies, they tend to adopt discourses relating to an ideal feminine bodily presentation and compare themselves unfavourably against this ideal. Although Irigaray and Kristeva appear to celebrate the mad body and its gestures as an expression of feminine syntax, they nevertheless make a valuable contribution to the understanding of women's mental distress and its often non-verbal expression. In these terms, mental health practitioners need to make room to decipher the meanings inherent in the body and its expression, particularly while working with women mental health patients.

## Klein, the body and psychosis

I will now outline the work of Melanie Klein and ways in which her work illuminates how defence mechanisms including 'splitting', 'introjection', 'projection' and 'projective identification' operate in the development of a sense of identity in babies. Klein also discusses how these early mechanisms can also form the basis of psychosis in adults. In addition, I will highlight ways in which the body of the infant and its primary carer are a dominant feature in Klein's discussions of these early mechanisms and her revision of Freud's theory of the Oedipus complex.

### Mother as central

Klein, who was born in 1882, and allegedly a rather strict and controlling mother,[2] brought about a major change within psychoanalysis and its previous focus on the father as central figure in an infant's development. Klein challenged this emphasis by focusing upon the importance of the mother, and, in particular, the mother's body. Klein practically ignores the 'social' interactions between the mother and infant as well as the 'real' environment.[3] What takes precedence for Klein, is the infant's fantasies about the mother's body.

### The Oedipus complex

In her 1928 paper 'Early Stages of the Oedipus Conflict' (in Mitchell 1986), Klein proposed that the Oedipus complex occurred earlier in life than Freud had suggested. Contrary to Freud, Klein suggested that the infant's Oedipus inclinations are released in connection with the frustrations the child experiences during weaning. These manifest themselves at the end of the first, and at the beginning of the second year of life and are then reinforced during the process of toilet training. For Klein, the Oedipus complex takes place during the oral and anal phases of development and not solely in the phallic phase as maintained by Freud. Klein states that during the oral 'sadistic' phase, which she claims is motivated by the biological death drive, the infant experiences a strong desire to bite and devour the mother in retaliation for her seemingly depriving the infant of food. During the anal sadistic phase, the infant perceives its mother as depriving it of its faeces. In addition it equates the mother's faeces with possible future brothers and sisters and with the father's penis. Consequently, the infant desires to rob the mother of her faeces. This is what Klein refers to as the 'femininity phase' in both sexes. In the boy, as well as wishing to attack his mother anally, he also experiences oral sadistic phantasies towards his mother's womb that he perceives as containing his father's penis.

Klein considers that the experiences of the two sexes further diverge as they enter the genital phase of development. She asserts that both sexes have an inherent unconscious knowledge of their sex organs (Doane and Hodges 1992: 12). The boy has up to now orally and anally hated his mother. This hatred causes him anxiety lest she retaliate by attacking him. According to Klein, the boy innately 'knows' the penetrative function of his penis and he now begins to genitally desire his mother. In addition his inherent unconscious knowledge of his possession of a penis influences his decision towards choosing his love object. However, his pre-genital oral and anal impulses are still very intense and the extent to which the boy attains genital eroticism will depend on his tolerance of his pre-genital anxiety. Klein states that, if the boy's hate for his mother is very intense, he may cling to his pre-genital impulses. The outcome of this process will influence his future relations with women.

In Klein's estimation, the girl carries her innate receptive aim from the oral to the genital phase. She also transfers her primary libidinal object from her mother to her father. This process is partly initiated by the girl's envy and hatred of her mother for taking the father's penis into her body. Due to her phantasised attacks on the mother, the girl also fears her mother's retaliation on her own sexual and reproductive capacity. However, the oral and anal deprivations experienced by the girl constitute the main reason for her turning away from the mother as her desired love object. These deprivations are also responsible for the girl's identity as hetero-sexual. She looks to her father to satisfy and repair previous deprivations by her mother. For Klein, it is the deprivations associated with the mother's breast, not her inferiority in lacking a penis as maintained by Freud, that is the cause of the girl turning towards her father and to her subsequent heterosexuality. Furthermore, according to Klein, it is the girl's wish to internalise the father's penis and to receive a child from him that 'precedes the wish to possess a penis of her own' (Klein in Segal 1992: 97). I will now turn to Klein's practise of play technique from which she formulated her object-relations theory.

### Play technique

Klein's analysis of young children led to the development of her object-relations theory. She used a play technique in which she provided children with small toys including dolls, containers, scissors, paper and pencils. Klein considered that she could gain access to the unconscious world of children and consequently decipher meanings behind their displays of aggression and anxiety. In her paper, 'The Psycho-analytic Play Technique' (1955), Klein states:

> Aggressiveness is expressed in various ways in the child's play, either directly or indirectly. Often a toy is broken or, when the child is more aggressive, attacks are made with knife or scissors on the table or on

pieces of wood; water or paint is splashed about and the room generally becomes a battlefield.

(Klein in Mitchell 1986: 41)

Klein emphasised that such aggressive attacks are directed towards the body of the mother or the primary carer.

In *The Psycho-Analysis of Children* (1997), Klein describes a three-year-old child called Trude. This child was neurotic and had a strong fixation on her mother. Trude's interaction with the small toys gave Klein insight into her expressions of anxiety. Trude insisted that flowers from a vase were removed and, having put a little toy man in a cart, hurled him out again inflicting abuse upon him. She demanded that a man wearing a high hat in her picture book be taken out, and stated that the cushions in the room had been thrown into disarray by a dog. Klein interpreted these actions as representing Trude's wish to do away with her father's penis. These toys – the cart, vase, cushion and picture book – were used by Trude to express her anxiety and therefore represented her mother's body thrown into disorder.

Due to external circumstances, Trude's analysis with Klein was interrupted but she returned after six months. On her return, she expressed her aggression towards her mother's body more vehemently. Trude insisted that it was night and both she and Klein had to go to sleep. She stole up to Klein, simulating the act of stabbing Klein in the throat, burning her, throwing her into the courtyard and giving her to a policeman. Klein further interpreted Trude's actions and concluded that she wished to look inside her mother's body and take out the faeces (which to Trude represented children). These wishes to attack her mother's body made Trude fearful, but by revealing them to Klein through play, she was able to bring them under conscious control. I will now discuss Klein's object-relations theory that stemmed from her findings using her play technique.

### Phantasies

According to Klein, the infant from birth relates to the breast and other objects in phantasy. The use of the word 'phantasy' rather than 'fantasy' was adopted by Klein to indicate unconscious rather than conscious fantasies. By observing her own son, Erich, at the ages of four and five, Klein emphasised that he related to the external world through phantasies that were influenced by his own psychical state. In a content mood, he saw Klein as a princess he wanted to marry. In contrast, when he was angry, he perceived Klein as a poisoning, threatening witch. According to Klein, the infant's phantasies often involve doing something to somebody who is outside and distinct from the self. This object may be part of the self that has been separated off. Klein proposed that children feel guilt as a result of such phantasies. Richard, one of the children she observed, had phantasies of attacking and damaging his father as a result of jealous rivalry. Richard became very upset when his father actually did fall down and become ill. He appeared to perceive this event as confirmation that his aggressive feelings could really cause severe damage.

### Objects as body parts

Klein emphasised that the infant's early experience of the world centres around its relationship to objects that can be perceived as inside or outside of itself. These objects are related to through unconscious phantasy and are motivated by the bodily instinctive drives of the infant, namely the oral, anal and genital drives. Unlike Freud, Klein did not believe the infant experiences these instincts in stages, but moves from one to the other following no particular sequence. For the infant, according to Klein, its objects are parts of its own and its parents' bodies. Klein stated that body parts including the breast, penis and so forth, are objects that can be either wholly or partially cathected. Klein stated that the phantasised relationship the infant has with its parents' bodies is often revealed through play.

The children she observed would simulate the actions of eating paper or drinking from a tap. Klein interpreted these actions as indicating an infant's wish to take inside parts of its parents' bodies, which the child experiences concretely, as Klein explains: 'The baby, having incorporated his parents, feels them to be live people inside his body in the concrete way in which deep unconscious phantasies are experienced – they are, in his mind, "internal" or "inner" objects' (Klein in Mitchell 1986: 148). It is the internalisation of these objects that are a source of anxiety and emotional ambivalence for the infant. Klein states that these early experiences of anxiety are necessary for the infant to form an identity of its own. For this to occur, the infant has to experience two psychical events. Klein does not refer to these as stages, but rather as 'positions' which she called 'paranoid–schizoid' and the 'depressive'. Within these positions, the infant has to negotiate a number of defence mechanisms including 'splitting', 'introjection', 'projection' and 'projective identification'.

### Splitting

The process of splitting describes how the infant keeps the nurturing, good breast as quite distinct from the dangerous, bad breast. When the infant is in a state of bliss following a feed, it introjects a 'good' breast inside. This has to be kept safe from the bad breast that is also introjected by the infant as bad when it is feeling distressed and hungry. This process continues and the internalised bad object is experienced as so dangerous and painful that the infant has to split off this part of itself and project it onto external objects. Consequently, in the infant's world, other people are experienced as dangerous as they contain split off and projected parts of the infant's self.

### The paranoid–schizoid position

The paranoid–schizoid position occurs in the first three months when the infant is fused with the mother and is fixated upon its oral capacities for gaining pleasure by feeding from the breast. The infant will introject or take inside the good, nurturing breast. This is necessary for the infant's development, as she explains in 'Notes on Some Schizoid Mechanisms': 'This first internal good object acts as a focal point in the ego. It counteracts the processes of splitting and dispersal, makes for cohesiveness and integration, and is instrumental in building up the ego' (Klein in Mitchell 1986: 181).

Klein states that this experience of love is the result of a life instinct or drive. She also added another dimension to this process that involves the aggressive, sadistic phantasies of the infant towards the breast. When the infant is very hungry it experiences extreme bodily discomfort and feels that the object with which it is fused, the breast, is responsible for this discomfort. The infant is totally dependent upon the body of the mother and experiences destructive phantasies towards her, as Klein describes: 'From the beginning the destructive impulse is turned against the object and is first expressed in phantasised oral-sadistic attacks on the mother's breast, which soon develop into onslaughts on her body by all sadistic means' (ibid.: 177). Klein also describes how the infant uses other parts of its body or the mother's body in its attack.

There are also anal wishes whereby the infant wishes to expel harmful excrement from its own body and place it into the mother. The infant wishes to rob the mother's body of its good contents and get inside her body to control it from the inside. Following Freud, Klein asserts that such sadistic attacks on the mother's body are a result of an innate death drive. As a result of these sadistic phantasies, the infant introjects the bad breast into itself. However, to protect its ego from extreme anxiety it attempts to get rid of this badness and projects the badness out towards to an external object. The external breast now becomes the source of badness and threatens annihilation. The infant now fears, according to Klein, being devoured or having its internal organs scooped out by this external object.

### Projective identification

Another mechanism that runs parallel to splitting and which is also used by the infant within the paranoid–schizoid position is that of projective identification. Juliet Mitchell describes this process as occurring when, 'the ego projects its feelings into the object which it then identifies with, becoming like the object which it has already imaginatively filled with itself' (Mitchell 1986: 20). The infant attempts to deal with its destructive feelings by disowning them and placing them into something else. Consequently, infants fear their destruction coming at them from the outside, usually in the form of the devouring breast. Segal in *Melanie Klein*, quotes Ernest Jones' description of a small boy who upon observing his mother breastfeeding his new born brother, exclaimed while pointing at her breast: 'That's what you bit me with' (Jones in Segal 1992: 36).

## The depressive position

According to Klein, the infant's phantasised attacks on the mother's body eventually bring about feelings of guilt. At about three to six months the infant enters what Klein refers to as the depressive position. The infant experiences loss of the good breast and guilt about its destructive phantasies against it. Klein describes how the infant has internalised the good breast which has provided it with milk, love and security: 'All these are felt by the baby to be lost, and lost as a result of his own uncontrollable greedy and destructive phantasies and impulses against his mother's breasts' (Klein in Mitchell 1986: 148).

Within this position, the infant can begin to internalise the mother as a whole object that is comfortably both good and bad. In order for this to occur, the infant has to be able to repair the external world and its own damaged internal objects. With the internalisation of good objects and the experience of loving feelings the infant can restore a complete good enough mother and abandon feelings of annihilation, as Klein states: 'Along with the increase in love for one's good and real objects goes a greater trust in one's capacity to love and a lessening of the paranoid anxiety of the bad objects' (ibid.: 144). This position also marks the infant's successful separation from its mother.

There are two defences that occur within the depressive position, namely, denial and omnipotence. Denial occurs when the infant experiences and negates both dependence and ambivalent feelings towards the mother. Omnipotence involves the feelings of mastery and contempt that hide the distress associated with the loss of the mother, and in addition the endings of phantasised control over her. In the depressive position, anxiety results in depression rather than a desire to attack or fear of being attacked. At best, in this position, the infant can now begin to own its feelings and accept reality.

## The psychoses

As well as focusing upon the infant's relationship to its mother's body thereby attributing much importance to the role of the mother in early life,

Klein also brought about another theoretical shift in psychoanalysis. Freud and other analysts focused mainly on hysteria and the neuroses, Klein's emphasis upon the infant's early phantasised relations with internal and external objects brought about a better understanding of the mechanisms involved in the psychoses, as Klein herself states at the end of her paper, 'The Psycho-Analytic Play Technique': 'The fuller understanding of the earliest stages of development, of the role of phantasies, anxieties and defences in the emotional life of the infant has also thrown light on the fixation points of adult psychosis' (ibid.: 54).

Klein stated that every infant has destructive impulses towards its mother's body and these take the form of oral sadistic and anal sadistic attacks. She also states that the infant experiences defences of the ego including splitting, denial of inner and outer reality, the stifling of emotion and anxieties associated with being poisoned and devoured. Klein asserts, therefore, that all infants pass through a psychotic phase that is overcome with entry into the depressive position. She found, however, that these mechanisms were particularly intense in a number of children she analysed and she concluded that such children were suffering from childhood schizophrenia. Klein found that these children experienced intense fears about the retaliation of their aggressive impulses from others and that this was the basis or fixation point for the later development of psychosis in adults.

Klein describes 'Erna' a child of six, as suffocating and dominating her mother. Erna's mother, upon describing her daughter, exclaimed: 'She swallows me up'. Erna's symptoms began when she witnessed her parents having sex. In her analysis with Klein, Erna revealed how she felt rage towards her mother for giving her father all her attention. Erna split her objects and projected bad feelings into external figures. She revealed through play analysis with Klein her fears of persecutory retaliation. A toy man and woman represented a teacher and a mistress who were giving children lessons in good manners. Initially, Erna described the children as polite and good, but then they attacked the teacher and the mistress, trampling upon them and roasting them. In describing her analysis of Erna, Klein states how she underwent torments and humiliations from Erna and in addition, 'if anyone in the game treated me kindly, it generally turned out that the kindness was only simulated. The paranoiac traits showed in that I was constantly spied upon, people divided my thoughts' (Klein in Hinshelwood 1991: 408).

Klein states that if early sadistic impulses and defence mechanisms are very intense, the infant cannot work through the paranoid–schizoid position. Subsequent entry into the depressive position is also impeded which can result in psychosis, as described by Rosalind Minsky: 'the depressive position has been so unsuccessfully negotiated that one or other of the defences takes over and dominates over other forms of communication' (1996: 89). These other defences include projection, introjection, denial and omnipotence. Psychosis is therefore dominated by phantasies and defence mechanisms in which the result is a loss of reality. Klein states that in psychosis, the excessive splitting of the ego threatens to weaken it. The individual takes flight into an idealised internal object that serves to damage the ego further. The ego is consequently overwhelmed by its inner objects and cannot incorporate them into itself. In addition, the ego cannot take back in itself what it has previously projected outwards.

### Symbol-formation and psychosis

In her paper, 'The Importance of Symbol Formation in the Development of the Ego' (in Mitchell 1986), Klein discusses the importance of symbol formation in early development, and reveals how this process is hindered in psychosis. Murray Jackson defines symbols or symbol formation as necessary to all mental functioning: 'the ability to create symbolic *representations* of the external world and to develop the capacity for abstract conceptual thinking' (2001: 340). According to Jackson, in psychosis, the symbol is experienced as the thing symbolised and therefore thinking is concrete. In other words, the symbol is not a representation of a thing, but *is* the thing.

The psychoanalyst Hanna Segal offers examples of concrete thinking in the discussion of her work with psychotic patients. One patient brought into the consulting room a wooden stool he seemed acutely embarrassed by as if it was his faeces. Another patient, when asked why he had stopped playing the violin, described his fear at being seen to masturbate in public. This patient therefore experienced the violin and his penis as the same thing (Segal 1981: 104).

Klein's understanding of symbol formation involves focus upon the anxiety resulting from the infant's sadistic attacks on the mother's body. Anxieties about retaliation from attacked objects normally enable the infant to transfer phantasies and anxiety to new objects (or symbols) other than people or body parts, in order to escape the perceived danger. Klein offers an example of this when she describes a child who can understand that the toy he has just damaged only *represents* his brother, and he would not actually attack his real brother. This process, in Klein's view, is essential in enabling the child to form symbols. She states that in psychosis there is lack of not only affect, but in symbol formation.

Klein offers a case study of a boy named Dick, which highlights the lack of symbol formation in psychosis. Dick was four when Klein began his analysis. He was unable to form any attachment to his mother or wet-nurse, neither of whom showed him any affection. Dick himself expressed no emotion and refused to eat. His bodily movements were unco-ordinated and awkward and he was unable to hold implements such as scissors or tools. Even when he received more emotional attention from his grandmother and another nurse, he appeared not to take this in, and he still would only eat mashed up food.

Dick revealed to Klein through play analysis that he was so terrified of his own destructiveness that attachment to others was impossible for him. In speaking, he used a few words incorrectly and made some meaningless sounds and noises. It seemed to Klein that Dick had no wish to make himself understood. He expressed very little interest in the toys provided by Klein but did appear interested in door handles and doors, and the opening and shutting of them. Klein interpreted this fascination as Dick's perception of his mother's body. The door concretely stood for the way in and out of her body. The door handles stood for his father's penis and his own.

Through play, Dick began to reveal that parts of his body – penis, urine and faeces – stood for objects with which he wanted to attack his mother. Klein found that he feared actual retaliation from his father's penis for attacks on his mother. According to Klein, this curtailed his ability to create symbols. Dick, in Klein's view, had identified with the attacked object and he had consequently formed a defence against sadism. Klein states: 'The ego had ceased to develop phantasy life and to establish a relation with reality' (Klein in Mitchell 1986: 101). Dick was indifferent to the objects around him and their representations and meaning. Therefore, he experienced the world in concrete terms. Klein concluded that Dick was severely psychotic due to his lack of affect and inability to form symbols, his defences against his sadistic impulses towards his mother and his inability to tolerate anxiety. As a result of these, the development of his ego was impeded.

### The body in Klein's theories

Emphasis upon the body, then, appears to be a dominant factor within many of Klein's theories relating to early development. She appears to consider both the biological body and the body that represents both terrifying and nurturing phantasised objects. In her discussion of the development of the Oedipus complex, Klein appears to largely consider the body as biological. In her explanation of gender difference, for example, she states that the infant appears to possess biologically given inherent knowledge of its sexual organs. The girl, according to Klein, knows she has a vagina and therefore follows the road of femininity. The boy also appears to inherently 'know' he is in possession of a penis and takes up a masculine position. In her discussion of the infant's sadistic attacks on the mother's breast, Klein states that these stem from the biologically given death drive or instinct, theorised by Freud. In contrast, the loving feelings the baby experiences towards its mother's breast stem, according to Klein, from the life drive. These two biological instincts are in conflict with one another.

In her discussion of objects with which the infant relates in early life, Klein tends to consider the body as representative of something beyond physicality or biology. The infant's body and that of its mother stand as 'objects' rather than mere biological bodies. Klein describes the ways in which the infant has to negotiate its sense of identity within this world of objects that can be both devouring and terrifying, or nurturing and comforting. She focuses upon the infant's sense of what is both inside and outside its body and, more specifically, its relationship to the body of its mother.

In her emphasis upon symbol formation, she states that in psychosis objects literally stand for things, not as representations of things. In her case study of Dick, his penis, urine and so forth, concretely stood for the objects with which he attacked his mother's body. These were not felt in terms of phantasy, nor were his terrible fears of literal attack on him by his father's penis. This understanding may be useful in understanding the bodily experiences of psychotic people. The objects around them are often felt concretely or literally as aspects of themselves or their bodies. I relate these ideas to some of the patients I observe in Chapter 8.

### Concluding Klein

In conclusion, it is clear that Klein's theory of object-relations provides an understanding of ways in which the body is experienced in psychosis. According to Klein, in psychosis, there is regression to a primitive state where the infant internalises bad objects, namely, the body parts of its parents and projects them out onto external objects which are also in the form of its parents' bodies. Subsequently, the infant fears persecution from outside as occurs in the case of the person with psychosis who believes that others are putting thoughts into them, taking their thoughts out, or controlling them from the outside world or invading them.

As Klein states, the psychotic ego is severely fragmented so the individual cannot feel rooted in a complete 'self' or body. She appears to state that the process of projection, so vehemently carried out by an individual with psychosis, seems to begin from the body that is then transferred to the mind. The individual projects out bad parts of the self into eternal objects and then, through a process of introjection, fears outside control of them within. Klein adds: 'This may lead to the fear that not only the body but also the mind is controlled by other people in a hostile way' (Klein in Mitchell 1986: 185). Consequently, the individual is unable to introject good objects, which brings about further splitting, anxiety and withdrawal. In her emphasis on symbol formation, Klein proposes that these defence mechanisms in the psychotic person are felt concretely. Outside objects are literally felt as part of the self and there is a blurring between what is inside and outside. I will now turn to the post-Kleinian work of Wilfred Bion.

## Bion: thinking, frustration and psychosis

Wilfred Bion develops Klein's emphasis upon symbol formation. I will now briefly outline his contributions to the understanding of symbol forma- tion, or rather the lack of it, in psychosis. I consider that his theories also add to an understanding of the body in psychosis. I return to the work of Bion in the next chapter where I discuss the psychoanalytic concepts of transference and countertransference.

In his theory of thought processes, Bion states that raw sense data is made up of the individual's emotional experience and sensations from internal and external sources. Bion suggests that in order for an individual to think and give meaning to their experience of these sensations, they need to transform them into what he refers to as 'alpha elements'. Accord- ing to Bion, alpha elements provide the psyche with 'the material for dream thoughts and hence the capacity to wake up or go to sleep, to be conscious or unconscious' (1993: 115). Bion suggests that alpha function is neces- sary for dreaming, attention and the passing of judgement, as Joan and Neville Symington point out: 'A painful emotion, if acted upon by alpha function, is transformed into dream images and abstracted into thought' (1996: 62).

If the transformation of raw sense data into alpha elements fails to occur, then they remain as unassimilated 'beta elements'. These are made up of accumulated raw sense data. As an example of this, Bion offers the example of 'word-salad' in schizophrenic patients, which refers to a sequence of unconnected words. According to Bion, these impressions and sensations are experienced at the physiological level of pleasure or pain. He suggests that the raw sense data is processed by evacuation or in Kleinian terms as 'projective identification', rather than thinking. This evacuation process is frequently carried out as anxiety-driven activity. A patient, for example, states she does not have to get up to go to the toilet at night because she has had a dream. Thus, she is able to hold in her sensations by the dream and not evacuate them (Bion 1996).

Sensations are felt as things because they are not processed by thought and are got rid of as if they were things. Bion suggests that evacuation occurs through the body and uses the examples of grimacing or elbow rubbing. He states that the person cannot 'transform the experience so he can store it mentally . . . it is felt as a "thing" – lacking any quality we attribute to thought and verbal expression' (1992: 180). He states that this process is apparent in patients with schizophrenia. In his work with disturbed patients, Bion observed there were undigested fragments in the patient's speech rather than complete images. He also noticed that such patients have a limited capacity for dreaming.

In his paper, 'Notes on the Theory of Schizophrenia' (in Bion 1993), Bion states the difficulty the schizophrenic experiences in forming symbols, substantives and verbs. The difficulties in speech in schizophrenia are often referred to in psychiatric textbooks. An example is: 'speech may be poor in quantity and content, often eliciting vagueness' (Thompson and Mathias 2000: 180). However, there is rarely any analysis of why this happens. Bion suggests, following Klein, that such difficulties in speech are due to severe splitting mechanisms. He gives the example of a patient with schizophrenia who states a series of associations separated by spaces of four or five minutes, but none of which connect together. For Bion, this process – or lack of integration – makes language unavailable as a mode of thought. He argues that in order to effectively form symbols the individual has to be able to grasp complete and whole objects, and move on from the paranoid–schizoid position into the depressive position where there is an integration of previous splits. Bion suggests that in schizophrenia, the person will utilise language as a mode of action rather than thought. In his work with schizophrenic patients, Bion concluded that feelings in such patients are felt concretely as 'things'. In speech, words are experienced as objects or things, rather than as symbols for objects.

Bion suggests that the capacity for thought is also accompanied by the capacity for frustration. He gives the example of the baby's experience of a no-breast. This can be internalised and thought about and thus tolerated. If the capacity for frustration is lacking, then the breast is internalised as a bad object. What should be a thought becomes a bad object that the person attempts to get rid of. Bion suggests another aspect of the schizophrenic personality is a hatred of reality because the person fears the split off and persecutory aspects of it and consequently there is fear of attack from outside, or from 'bizarre objects', as Bion refers to them. According to Bion, there is also a resistance against the possible integration of these split off parts, such as in the analytic situation. He suggests that the analyst must translate the data he or she observes into a tolerable idea. I shall return to this point in the next chapter, where I discuss Bion and countertransference. I will now discuss the work of R.D. Laing and his understanding of the body in psychosis.

## Laing: the body as false self

Laing, a rather controversial figure to say the least, was born in 1927, studied medicine after leaving school, and specialised in neurology and psychiatry. After working in a British Army psychiatric unit, he eventually became a senior registrar in Glasgow, and then worked at the Tavistock Clinic in London, and began training as a psychoanalyst. After arriving in London, Laing published his first book *The Divided Self* (1969). This book proved to be a success. Following *The Divided Self*, Laing went on write other books including *Self and Others* (1961), *Sanity, Madness and the Family* (1964) and *The Politics of Experience* (1967).

Laing explored ways in which the notions of 'madness' and 'normality' are constructed, and questioned the value systems upon which these concepts are based. He also explored psychological violence within the family as instrumental in bringing about madness in individuals. Laing became associated with the anti-psychiatry movement, which set out to challenge existing concepts of mental illness, and to establish therapeutic communities as an alternative to hospitalisation. These communities set out to exclude both doctors and established psychiatric treatments for those with mental distress. For the purposes of this thesis, I will focus on *The Divided Self.* In this book, Laing explores the experience of psychosis and suggests it involves the individual experiencing a splitting between their 'true' or 'real' self, and the 'false' self or 'personality', centred in the body.

People with psychosis, in Laing's estimation, need to be understood from an existential perspective. When interacting with such people, states Laing, we have to be aware of our own psychotic potential, in order to discover how they experience themselves and the world around them. It is not enough solely to focus on the symptoms the patient presents. We have to realise his or her existential position: 'One cannot love a conglomeration of "signs of schizophrenia". No one *has* schizophrenia, like having a cold ... The schizophrenic has to be known without being destroyed' (1969: 34). Therefore, according to Laing, schizophrenia is a way of experiencing the world and if we reject the terminology used to describe the condition, such as that found within psychiatric textbooks, and listen to the language of the schizophrenic, we would then understand and communicate with them better.

### Ontological insecurity

A state of ontological security refers to the way an individual experiences the world without fear of annihilation. A sane person will experience his or her being as real, integrated and alive. The inner self is therefore experienced as worthy, substantial and consistent. In terms of the body, the sane individual will experience his or her identity, according to Laing, 'as spatially co-extensive with the body' (ibid.: 41). Psychoses may develop, however, when the individual experiences ontological insecurity, which develops early in life. In this case, according to Laing, the individual will experience a lack of personal cohesiveness and integration. They will also feel divorced from their body. Outside reality is felt to persecute and threaten annihilation. They may feel turned to stone and without autonomy. To deal with their inner deadness, they may also turn other people to stone so they will not impinge.

Laing describes three states of anxiety associated with ontological insecurity. 'Engulfment' describes a fear of relatedness and relations with others threatening the individual's lack of inner integration and identity. 'Implosion' refers to outside reality being experienced as threatening to intrude and explode one's being. 'Petrification' describes feeling turned to stone by terror, or turning others to stone, or dead things. 'Depersonalisation' describes a process whereby the individual no longer feels responsive to others' feelings, and considers that others are not responsive to their feelings.

### The self as unembodied

Most individuals experience a state of being detached from their bodies at certain times, and this can be beneficial in certain circumstances. With reference to this, Laing offers an example of a man who is attacked in an alleyway. The attackers hit the man with a cosh, which stuns him momentarily. The man, feeling detached from his body during the attack, states that, although the attackers hit him (his body), *he* was not harmed. His body and self were therefore dissociated. Laing states that a sense of embodiment, or being in one's body, means that the individual is 'fully implicated in his body's desires, needs, acts, is subject to the guilt attendant on such desires, needs and actions' (ibid.: 68). A feeling of being in one's body, therefore, according to Laing, does not fully protect the individual from outside threat, fear or insecurity.

Laing describes psychosis, by contrast, in terms of detaching one's 'true' or 'inner' unembodied self, from one's outer embodied 'false self' or 'personality'. In this case, as Laing describes, *'The body is felt more as one object among other objects in the world than as the core of the individual's own being'* (ibid.: 69; italics in original). The body, therefore, takes on a separate persona or a mask and Laing suggests that this aspect of the individual may take the form of various impersonations. The false self may be felt as a threat to the inner or true self. In this sense, the individual, according to Laing, experiences a sense of being 'self-conscious' whereby they feel under the observation of the 'other'. The process of creating the false self is an attempt to preserve and protect the inner self.

In the form of a case study, Laing presents 'David', who took on an impersonation of his mother. He was inseparable from her and had always been a 'good' child. When his mother died, David took over her role by cooking the meals, buying food and looking after his father. He also revealed an interest in her keenness for embroidery and interior decoration. David, throughout his childhood, had been fond of playing certain roles in front of the mirror, and these roles were always female characters. He would dress in his mother's clothes and found himself playing the part of a woman by talking, walking and thinking in ways he thought a woman might talk, walk or think. Laing suggests that David experienced his mother as a potentially engulfing figure inside of him. Taking on her persona, according to Laing, was David's way to 'arrest the womanish part that threatened to engulf not only his actions but even his "own" self as well, and to rob him of his much cherished control and mastery of his being' (ibid.: 72).

Laing states that the false self can be felt by the individual as a source of protection of the true, inner self that is hidden from the world and reality. However, he states this does not work and the split between the true and false selves increases. The separate parts of the self work independently of each other. The speech patterns of the false self appear affected and unreal, as if foreign. Laing suggests that the schizophrenic 'symptom' of 'word-salad' (muddled up words) is an example of this. The true self, protected from destruction, actually experiences terror, guilt and despair. Laing suggests that the true self, which Laing refers to as the shut-up self, wishes to be alive and get inside life again, but cannot find the means to do this.

In the final chapter of *The Divided Self*, Laing presents the case of a schizophrenic woman named Julie, who had been hospitalised for nine years. She is presented as withdrawn and inaccessible. This woman hallucinated and appeared to make no sense verbally. She refers to herself as the 'occidental sun' and as 'Mrs Taylor'. After interviewing her family, Laing suggests how this woman's presentation begins to make sense in terms of her lived experience. Her mother, for instance, was ambivalent about having Julie and claimed she both wanted and did not want her. The pregnancy turned out to be accidental and Julie's mother actually wanted a son. Consequently Julie's descriptions of herself as 'occidental sun' made sense. She felt tailor-made (Mrs Taylor) by her mother. Laing emphasises the point that he was able to develop a rapport with this patient and therefore gained insight into her psychotic presentation. Julie was caught up in her attack on her mother and her mother's counter-attack. Furthermore, there was an absence in her world of someone who could cherish and make sense of her experience and point of view.

### Concluding Laing

Laing's descriptions of the split occurring in people with psychosis, provides valuable insight into their inner experience cut off from their bodily experience. The inner self transcends the world and is therefore kept safe against annihilation. The embodied persona represents an attempt to protect the inner self and arrest the fear of engulfment. The body, then, is felt as a persecuting figure, yet it is also a potential refuge. The personae patients take on in the form of delusions, whether they are God or Spartacus, serve to have particular meanings for that individual. Laing thereby reinforces an appreciation of, and the need to understand, the lived experience of people with psychosis.

## Conclusion

In this chapter, I have discussed the work of theorists who apply their concepts to an understanding of the psychical and bodily experiences of people with psychosis. Schilder contends that the person with psychosis lacks a sense of being in, or owning, their body due to an absence of libidinal investment in it; Lacan considers the body image and psychosis in his mirror stage of ego formation; Irigaray and Kristeva state that women's suffering cannot be readily articulated in language and is, instead, expressed through the body and its gestures; Klein's concepts of the infant's experience of complex internal objects through processes of projection and introjection, are valuable in the conceptualisation of body image, identity and the self; Bion suggests that people with psychosis project out their sensations through their bodies rather than processing them by thinking; Laing proposes that people with psychosis experience a split between their true and false selves. The false self is experienced as embodied which serves to protect the true self from annihilation.

Many of these perspectives indicate some sort of disruption of the process of early development. For Lacan, the infant remains in the pre-imaginary stage where the body, and therefore the ego, is fragmented and uncoordinated. In Klein's estimation, the defensive mechanisms used by the infant in the paranoid–schizoid stage remain active into adulthood. Practitioners might observe that the people they care for are using such mechanisms defensively. We might be able to conclude that we can make sense of these mechanisms and that they do, in fact, have relevance in terms of the patient's relationships and experiences. In this way, we can understand our patients better. However, how might this increased understanding help patients? A woman patient, for instance, might say she has insects invading her body from outside and is very distressed by her symptoms. Is it that, as Bion suggests, she has expelled these painful thoughts from her mind or has experienced them at a physiological level and not as thoughts? What can we do as practitioners in these circumstances? As mental health practitioners we need to be able to bear somebody's distress and stay with them and this requires time and energy. By staying with people in their distress we can, perhaps, turn painful experiences into thoughts that can be better tolerated by the person. This requires us to think about the people we care for. However, in nursing practice we tend to be caught up with action and outcomes, rather than 'thinking'. Yet nurses are privileged in that they have the opportunity to spend quality time with their patients and therefore do have the opportunity to work therapeutically with them. I shall continue this discussion in Chapter 9.

I will now discuss the body of the practitioner. Attention to, and acknowledgement of, bodily responses in work with mentally distressed people, is a powerful means of understanding them better. In the next chapter I will discuss psychoanalytic concepts of transference, countertransference and body countertransference. I draw upon these concepts in discussing my findings in interacting with mental health patients, which I outline in Chapter 8.

# Chapter 7

# The practitioner's body

So far, I have focused upon the 'patient's body' in terms of its role in communicating mental distress, or more specifically, the life experiences of someone experiencing distress. In this chapter, I discuss the importance of the practitioner's body. In working with distressed people, we often experience responses that are both emotional and physical. Often it is difficult to make a distinction between these two responses. When we feel frightened, for example, we feel it in our bodies and we also 'think' about it. Attention to such responses belongs very much to the practice of psychoanalysis. In this chapter, I will outline the psychoanalytic understandings of transference, countertransference and body countertransference, and attempt to apply them to mental health practice.

By acknowledging, examining and making sense of their own emotional and physical responses to the bodily presentation of patients, mental health practitioners may better understand their patients' mental distress. For example, the anger and fear felt by staff towards a patient who neglects self-care may be helpful in revealing unconscious intentions on the part of the patient and possible causes of this in, for instance, fear. I will first consider the psychoanalytical concepts of transference and countertransference put forward by Freud. I will then discuss subsequent post-Freudian theories.

## Freud on transference and countertransference

The psychoanalytic concept of transference refers to the way in which unconscious ideas and feelings are placed onto external objects and persons. The psychoanalytic writers Laplanche and Pontalis characterise transference as involving the re-emergence of infantile wishes: 'In the transference, infantile prototypes re-emerge and are experienced with a strong sense of immediacy' (1988: 455). For example, a patient may have repressed into their unconscious an early forbidden sexual wish. Psychoanalytic technique encourages past childhood conflicts to re-emerge using the process of free association. This enables a patient's repressed desire to resurface so that they transfer this desire onto the analyst.

Freud's writings on transference show how his perspectives changed and developed over time. In his essay, *The Psychotherapy of Hysteria* (1895) Freud refers to transference as a 'false connection'. He describes how the hysterical symptoms in one of his female patients relate to a wish stemming from her past, which involved a male acquaintance taking the initiative to kiss her. Freud describes how within the psychoanalytic encounter, this patient had experienced a similar wish from him. This indicates how this wish was transferred onto Freud.

Freud also describes transference as an 'obstacle' that serves to reduce the likelihood of repressed contents being brought into consciousness. He stresses that transference onto the analyst by the patient most often occurs at the moment when there is a strong likelihood of important repressed material being exposed: 'the "obstacle" used not to appear directly as a result of my pressure, but I was always able to discover it if I took the patient back to the moment at which it had originated' (1895b: 303). In this context, transference can be seen to be a form of resistance.

It appears from these early writings that Freud did not fully formulate the concept of transference, and did not realise how crucial it was to address the transference if psychoanalysis was to be effective. Freud's treatment of his hysterical patient Dora in 1900, for example, shows that he does not consider psychoanalytic treatment as consisting of a transference relationship. In *Fragment of an Analysis of a Case of Hysteria*, Freud states: 'What are transferences? They are new editions or facsimiles of the impulses and phantasies which are aroused and made conscious during the progress of the analysis' (1905a: 116). Also, he concedes that the early termination of his analysis of Dora was due to his inability to fully comprehend the transference.

Freud further develops his theory of transference in his later writings and links it to his theory of the Oedipus complex, thus giving it an important place within the psychoanalytic encounter. In *The Dynamics of Transference* (1912) for example, Freud describes how adult sexuality is formed through experiences and influences from early life. These lead to a 'stereotype plate' (1912: 100) which, during the course of the person's life, is constantly repeated. During the process of individual development, a certain component of the impulses that determine the individual's erotic life will have undergone full psychical development. The remaining component is curtailed and consequently removed from conscious life and reality. This remaining component may be revealed within the individual's phantasy life, but may also be entirely unknown as it resides in the unconscious. Freud states that if in reality there is no satisfaction of an individual's need for love, the individual will encounter new people in their life 'with libidinal anticipatory ideas' (ibid.). Both the conscious and unconscious fragments of the individual's libido will serve to influence the formation of this attitude. Freud proceeds to describe how in the psychoanalytic encounter this process also takes place. This time the unsatisfied libidinal cathexis is directed to the analyst.

In Freud's estimation, patients' early relationship with their parents re-emerges within the psychoanalytic encounter and is 'lived out' in the transference. He stresses that the analyst can symbolise for the patient the 'imago'[1] of the father, the early relationship to the mother and the siblings. Laplanche and Pontalis describe the development of Freud's theory of transference as coinciding with the development of his theory of the Oedipus complex: 'All the way, the idea that transference actualises the essence of the childhood conflict is constantly gaining ground' (Laplanche and Pontalis 1988: 459).

In *The Dynamics of Transference*, Freud distinguishes between 'negative' and 'positive' transference. Positive transference constitutes affectionate and friendly feelings from the patient towards the analyst. He states that positive transference feelings can be further divided into those that are able to be included within the conscious life, and those that are unconscious. Negative transference constitutes hostile feelings that the patient transfers onto the analyst.

In his essay, 'Remembering, Repeating and Working-Through' (1914) Freud states that the patient often fails to remember past repressed conflicts, but rather acts them out and repeats this process. He argues that the patient does not 'remember' but reproduces the past through repeated actions: the 'compulsion to repeat'. Freud contends that the patient commences treatment exclaiming that they can remember nothing, thereby exhibiting this repetition. This inability to remember is a form of resistance. Freud examines the relation of this compulsion to repeat to resistance and transference: 'the transference is itself only a piece of repetition ... the repetition is a transference of the forgotten past not only onto the doctor but also on to all the other aspects of the current situation' (1914: 151). The patient, in his repetition repeats 'everything that has made its way from the sources of the repressed into his manifest personality' (ibid.). Freud states that the tool for curtailing the patient's compulsion to repeat and bringing about the process of remembering is in the technique of negotiating the transference.

Here, Freud introduces his concept of 'transference neurosis' that refers to an artificial neurosis upon which the manifestations of the transference are placed. The patient repeats their infantile conflicts in the transference and as Freud states: 'the transference thus creates an intermediate region between illness and real life through which the transition from the one to the other is made' (ibid.: 154). Here, it is clear that Freud perceives the psychoanalytic encounter as fundamentally a transference relationship. The patient's relationship to the analyst in the transference process has become the central focus. Freud concludes that the 'working-through' in the psychoanalytic encounter enables the patient to curtail the compulsion to repeat by the understanding and acceptance of previously repressed material. I shall now turn to Freud's work on countertransference.

Laplanche and Pontalis define the concept of countertransference as: 'The whole of the analyst's unconscious reactions to the individual analysand – especially to the analysand's own transference' (1988: 92). However, Freud alluded only briefly to the concept of the countertransference in his writings. In *The Future Prospects of Psycho-Analytic Therapy* (1910) for example, he describes countertransference as the result of the influence upon the analyst of the patient's unconscious feelings. Freud proposes that the analyst must be aware of such feelings and strive to overcome them. He states that, 'no psychoanalyst goes further than his own complexes and internal resistances permit' (1910: 145). Freud states that consequently, the analyst needs to undergo self-analysis while making observations on their patients. Therefore, the analyst becomes aware of his or her resistances and consequently become more receptive to the unconscious feelings that are transferred onto them by the patient. Freud warns that if this process does not occur in the analyst, then they should abandon the idea of being able to treat patients using the psychoanalytic technique.

Freud alludes to the concept of countertransference in 'The Disposition to Obsessional Neurosis' (1913). In this paper, he describes several different types of neurosis which have varying dispositions and which are formulated at different stages in life. He describes 'hysterical neurosis' as originating in earliest childhood, 'obsessional neurosis' originating between the ages of six to eight years, and 'paraphrenia' as beginning after puberty and during adult life. Freud describes a later neurosis – 'megalomania' – as characteristic of a turning away from objects, and difficulty in the transference process. He states that this form of neurosis originates in the auto-erotic and narcissistic stage of libidinal development prior to object choice.

Freud proceeds to present a case study of a woman who initially displays the symptoms of 'hysterical neurosis' and then 'obsessional neurosis'. She is happy until she learns that she is unable to have children by her husband whom Freud describes as 'the only object of her love' (1913: 320). Upon this realisation she becomes unwell with 'anxiety hysteria', which displays itself in her response to her frustration. She begins to have phantasies of seduction, which serve as an outlet for her wish for a child. The woman does everything she can to prevent her husband from guessing she has fallen ill as a result of her distress at being childless, of which he is the cause. Freud alludes to the occurrence of countertransference in this situation, by describing how the husband understands his wife's distress, despite all her efforts to conceal it from him. Freud explains this phenomenon by stating: 'I have good reason for asserting that everyone possesses in his own unconscious an instrument with which he can interpret the utterances of the unconscious in other people' (ibid.). Freud describes how the husband feels hurt in his realisation of his wife's distress, but does not reveal this to his wife. However, it displays itself neurotically when the husband, for the first time, fails in sexual intercourse with his wife. He then starts out on a journey. Believing that her husband is now impotent, the wife exhibits her first obsessional symptom the day before his return. She indulges in over-zealous washing and cleaning and endorses measures to prevent serious injury that she believes she has the potential to impose upon others. According to Freud, these displays of 'obsessional neurosis' are indicative of a sexual need resulting from the impotence of her husband.

In *Observations on Transference-Love* (1914), he describes how in the psychoanalytic situation, a phenomenon occurs whereby the patient falls in love with their doctor or analyst. Insisting upon addressing the patient as 'she' and the doctor as 'he', Freud describes that upon the termination of the analysis, the patient will repeat this process of falling in love with her second doctor and so forth. Freud proposes that both the doctor and the patient must reflect upon this process, which he describes as the foundation of psychoanalytic theory. He states that for the doctor, the transference of love by the patient is greatly valuable and insightful. Freud contends that the doctor has to be aware of countertransference feelings appearing in his own mind. The transference love must be perceived as an integral part of the analytic process and not as a result of any charms the doctor may possess.

If the doctor responds to his countertransference feelings evoked by the patient and returns her love, this would defeat the aims and purpose of the treatment. Freud stresses that the patient would have achieved success in acting out, repeating in reality what she should have just remembered. These memories would be kept within the domain of psychical events. Freud states that an actual love relationship would bring out 'all the inhibitions and pathological reactions of her erotic life, without there being any possibility of correcting them' (1914c: 166). Freud thus demonstrates that transference love is something integral to the analytic process and that the countertransference feelings evoked by this process must be kept in check by the analyst. I will now turn to Freud's discussion of transference and countertransference in relation to psychosis.

## Freud on psychosis and transference

As we have seen, Freud worked predominantly with patients suffering from neurosis and stated that the process of transference is less likely to occur when the patient has a psychotic illness. As Freud describes in his essay, 'Neurosis and Psychosis' (1924), among other things, psychotic people are generally unsuitable for analysis because of their incapacity to form 'a libidinal cathexis of real persons, which makes the emotional transference to the analyst possible' (Freud 1986: 560). Freud's considerations of psychosis can be divided into three main areas beginning with early works where he appears to concentrate on the role of defence in the production of psychotic symptoms in his essay, 'The Neuro-Psychoses of Defence' (1894). Second, he presents a case study of a paranoiac patient named Judge Schreber in 1911 and offers psychoanalytic interpretations, and third, Freud differentiates between neurosis and psychosis by examining the role of the ego and its relation with the id and the external world in writings including *The Loss of Reality in Neurosis and Psychosis* (1924). Although he claimed that people with psychosis were unable to form a transference onto their analyst, he nevertheless presents psychotic symptoms as meaningful in terms of the lived experience of the individual.

In 'The Neuro-Psychoses of Defence', Freud examines the role of defence in the production of certain symptoms belonging to both the neuroses (hysteria, phobias and obsessions) and psychoses (hallucinatory confusion). In neurosis an intolerable idea is repressed (and in the case of hysteria, for example, is transferred into a somatic symptom). In the case of 'hallucinatory confusion', the ego rejects an intolerable idea altogether as if it has never occurred. Freud states: 'from the moment at which this has been successfully done the subject is in a psychosis, which can only be classified as "hallucinatory confusion"' (1894: 58). Freud states that the intolerable idea is attached to reality, so the ego, to wholly detach itself from this idea, also has to perform this function. The detachment from reality brings about a hallucinatory state. Freud states that examples of these phenomena can be observed in the 'insane asylum'. A mother, for example, who has lost her child, as a form of defence creates a false reality and 'now rocks a piece of wood unceasingly in her arms' (ibid.: 60).

In *Psychoanalytic Notes on an Autobiographical Account of a Case of Paranoia* (1911), Freud presents a psychoanalytic interpretation of a paranoiac patient he never met, named Judge Schreber. Freud made an interpretation of Schreber by reading this patient's own account of his paranoid illness, *Memoirs of My Nervous Illness*, published in 1903. Schreber says in his account that a physician called Professor Flechsig treated him. Schreber initially appears to worship his physician but later refers to him as his persecutor. His illness begins with some hypochondriacal symptoms and a period of sleeplessness. Schreber expresses a fear that the end of the world will soon occur, and only he will remain. In addition, he believes that he is dead and rotting. Schreber describes how he would sit without moving for several hours and attempt to drown himself in the bath.

Schreber then develops religious delusions whereby he believes he is able to communicate with God and live in another world. Schreber perceives God as being made only of nerves. These nerves, referred to by Schreber as rays, are powerful and infinite and have the ability to create any kind of perceivable object. Schreber also accuses others of persecuting and harming him. He directs these delusions against his physician Flechsig who he refers to as a 'soul-murderer'. He also states a belief that his role in life is to 'redeem the world and to restore mankind to their lost state of bliss' (Freud 1911a: 16). He states that a vital component of this mission would consist of his being transformed into a woman. During this stage of his illness, Schreber describes bodily sensations involving his genitals being retracted into his body and transforming into female genitalia. He believes that a number of female nerves have been placed into his body from which will emerge a new race of men. This would result from impregnation from God's 'rays'. Schreber believes that this birth of a new race would enable him to have a natural death. He also suggests that God, for his own satisfaction, was insisting upon him becoming female. Schreber also believes the sun has the ability to speak in human language to him; the sun also stands in direct relation to God. However, Schreber often shouts abuse at the sun and seeks to shut it out.

Freud argues that Schreber's psychotic symptoms emerge from a passive homosexual desire for his father, and fear surrounding the threat of castration from him. He represses these feelings, projects them out and they return in the form of persecutory delusions. This, according to Freud, constitutes the paranoiac aspect of Schreber's illness. Freud basically asserts that the male paranoiac will deny his desire for another man. This potentially rather offensive and spurious suggestion has its useful points. Freud usefully demonstrates how the process of projection transforms feelings. The individual experiences the previously loved object as one he now hates. This hated object has now become a persecutor. The libido that was previously directed towards an external love object becomes detached. This detachment of the libido symbolises for Freud the process of regression. The libido attaches to the ego therefore aggrandising it. This means there is a regression to the stage of narcissism, whereby the person's only love object is his own ego. Freud refers to the work of Karl Abraham who specifies how psychotic people turn away from the external world. Hallucinations thus indicate the battle between regression and attempts to direct the libido back onto external objects.

Schreber initially directed his homosexual desire towards his physician, whom he initially worshipped, and this was later directed towards God. Therefore, the physician and God both symbolise Schreber's father (and it seems from Freud's account that following the early death of Schreber's father, his older brother took his father's place). Freud states that the sun is also a 'father-symbol'. These characters all become persecutory towards Schreber. After his recovery, Schreber seemed to boast of his ability to look at the sun with no difficulty and without being overly dazzled by it. The rays of God made up of nerve-fibres and spermatozoa symbolise a projection of Schreber's homosexual longings for his father.

Schreber's wishful phantasy of transforming into a woman is, according to Freud, a denied fear of castration from the father. Freud also connects this wishful phantasy to Schreber's reports that although he had a happy marriage, there were no children. According to Freud, the wish to transform himself into a woman indicated that Schreber desired the ability to have children successfully. Schreber's delusion that he would give birth to a new race of men and create another world, indicated for Freud, an escape from his situation of childlessness. In addition, Freud argues that this delusion is a way of repopulating the world derided from Schreber's narcissistic self-absorption.

In his essay, 'Neurosis and Psychosis' (1924), Freud differentiates between these two states. In the case of neurosis, the ego being dependent upon reality, represses the powerful force of the id. In psychosis, the ego under the influence of the id, withdraws from external reality. Freud thus states that in neurosis, reality is the dominant feature, whereas in psychosis it is the id. However, in *The Loss of Reality in Neurosis and Psychosis* (1924), Freud pinpoints that neurotic patients also appear to partake in a flight from reality. However, he argues that the flight from reality occurs when there is an attempt to find a compensation for the damaged or repressed id. In the case of psychosis, there is the withdrawal of the ego from reality (not from the id as is the case of neurosis) and an attempt to repair the damage done. At the expense of a restriction of reality, there is a new reality created. As Freud states: 'neurosis does not disavow the reality, it only ignores it; psychosis disavows it and tries to replace it' (1924b: 185). Previous 'memory-traces', 'judgements' and 'ideas' represented in the mind as reality and which are altered by new perceptions make for a new reality in the form of hallucinations. Freud suggests that these forms of a new reality are previously rejected and have forced themselves on the individual's consciousness. In both neurosis and psychosis, an attempt at reparation is unsuccessful. In neurosis, the repressed instinct fails at finding an effective substitute. In the case of psychosis, the creation of a new reality is never satisfactory. There is an attempt by the neurotic patient to replace a disagreeable reality with one that is more pleasant, which is achieved by phantasy. In psychosis, the imaginary external world attempts to replace the external reality.

We can conclude from Freud's writings on the mechanisms of psychosis outlined above, that psychotic patients may be considered as unsuitable for psychoanalytic treatment. There is a loss of external reality and the tendency to create a new reality while attaching certain secret meanings and significance to objects. The libidinal instincts become attached to the individual's own ego (narcissism) which means there is a severely reduced capacity for patients to form libidinal attachments to others. Consequently, as the libidinal attachments are directed inwards rather than outwards, this brings about a situation whereby the patient is less able to transfer feelings onto the analyst. However, Freud's psychoanalytic interpretations of psychosis provide us with a consideration that is not acknowledged within mainstream psychiatric thought. With its limited focus on symptoms and diagnostic category, and viewpoint that mental illness is predominantly caused by the imbalance or lack of brain chemicals, psychiatry tends to overlook the lived experiences of the patient. In the case of Schreber, Freud relates his psychotic symptoms to his lived experience. Thus, his symptoms are considered as symbols (for example, the sun as 'father-symbol') rather than just merely the outcome of a physiological disorder. I will now discuss theorists who consider that psychotic individuals can form a transference towards the analyst and are therefore suitable for analytic treatment.

## Klein and post-Kleinians on transference and countertransference

In *A Dictionary of Kleinian Thought*, R.D. Hinshelwood states that discussion of countertransference, 'underwent a remarkable metamorphosis in the 1950s' (1991: 255). It was the work of Klein that initiated theorists to discuss countertransference not as something to be overcome, but as a valuable tool in the analytic relationship. Such theorists in their writings on countertransference also specify that individuals with a psychosis can in fact form a transference onto the analyst but this differs to neurotic transference. These theorists have adopted the Kleinian concepts of projection, introjection and projective identification in exploring transference in patients with a psychosis. I will now turn to the work of these theorists beginning with Klein and her view of transference.

## Klein: projective identification and transference

In Chapter 6, where I discussed the body in psychosis, I outlined in detail Klein's use of the terms projection, introjection and projective identification. I will only describe them briefly here. In her paper, 'Notes on Some Schizoid Mechanisms' (1946), Klein describes projection as occurring due to an outward deflection of the death instinct. The ego, in order to overcome overwhelming anxiety, projects out or rids itself of badness. The perceived bad part of the self is projected out onto external objects. Introjection is the taking in of outside things. Klein states that this is also a defensive action involving the ego: 'Introjection of the good object is also used by the ego as a defence against anxiety' (Klein in Mitchell 1986: 181). Klein's use of the terms 'good object' or 'bad object' indicates that representation of internal and external objects are present in the infant's psyche from birth. The primary object of the infant in early life is the mother's breast. The infant relates to objects while experiencing an array of emotions including love, hatred, defensiveness and anxiety. Furthermore, these objects are related to in phantasy. One such example of this is the infant's experience of projective identification. The infant projects its badness onto the mother who, in turn, is identified with and experienced as the bad self. In phantasy, the infant during the paranoid–schizoid position will feel this external bad self as potentially persecutory towards it.

In her paper, 'The Origins of Transference' (1952), Klein argues that the material transferred on to the therapist originates in the primitive processes that the infant experiences from birth. The first anxiety is where the infant fears retaliation from the previously projected out parts containing the bad self. The infant undergoes a splitting process where objects are perceived in terms of either good or bad. Feelings of love and hate are clearly differentiated from each other. It is not until the occurrence of the depressive position that the ego begins to integrate. Aspects of love and hate, good and bad, become more synthesised. However, this brings about new anxiety whereby the infant perceives that its aggressive impulses against the bad breast may endanger the good, loved breast. According to Klein the infant fears its destruction towards the whole object: 'the infant feels he has destroyed or is destroying the whole object by his greed and uncontrollable aggression' (Klein in Mitchell 1986: 203).

Klein states that the processes of projection and introjection continue with the arrival of the Oedipus complex. New objects such as the father's penis take precedence over the mother's breast. With the acquiring of mental and physical skills and the integration of the ego, the infant will be able to form symbols. Accordingly, the transference of phantasies and emotions from one object to another will become possible. For Klein, early processes of splitting, projection, introjection and projective identification are repeated and accompanied by anxieties in adult life. These form the basis of material transferred onto the analyst. Through exploring the links between present and early life, the ego is strengthened and as Klein states, 'the phantastic aspects of objects lose in strength' (ibid.: 210).

Klein argues contrary to Freud, that schizophrenic patients do indeed form a transference onto the analyst. She states this is due to their use of projective defences stemming from early life, namely during the paranoid–schizoid position. Hinshelwood states that Klein does not discuss countertransference widely in her writings, but does acknowledge the importance of the therapist being aware of their unconscious in their work with children. In 'On Observing the Behaviour of Young Infants' (1955) for example, she states: 'If we are to understand the young infant ... we need not only greater knowledge but also a full sympathy with him, based on our unconscious being in close touch with his unconscious' (Klein *et al.* 1955: 237). I will now outline selected writings by Winnicott, Little, Bion, Rosenfeld and Searles who draw upon Klein's work in the understanding of transference and countertransference in working with people with psychosis.

## Winnicott: tolerating hate in the countertransference

In his 1947 paper 'Hate in the Countertransference', Donald Winnicott states that working with psychotic patients can provoke feelings of hate in those who work with them. He discusses the emotional burden that can be evident in the mental health nurse or the psychiatrist. For this understandable hate to be tolerated, according to Winnicott, it needs to be 'sorted out and conscious' (1947: 194). Those who work closely with people with psychosis, including the psychoanalyst, must explore the emotional development of the patient, in particular the early primitive stages, and explore the effects of the emotional burden upon the worker.

Winnicott defines what he refers to as the 'objective' countertransference, which constitutes the reactions or responses in the analyst to the behaviour of a patient. These are brought about by objective observation. Winnicott specifies that the analyst must be able, in their work with psychotic patients, to be able to study and make sense of their objective countertransference reactions. Such feelings, including those of objective hate, must be separated from unconscious hate stemming from the analyst's past and from their inner conflicts. This, according to Winnicott, justifies the view that analysts must undertake their own analysis to be able to work effectively with patients.

The psychotic patient, in the analytic situation, will experience a 'coincident love-hate' state of feeling, whereby affectionate and murderous feelings are intermingled. The analyst also needs to be aware of these emotions within him. The patient will only be able to appreciate in the analyst the feelings he is capable of experiencing. As Winnicott states, the person with psychosis may feel that the analyst 'is also only capable of the same crude and dangerous state of coincident love-hate . . . should the analyst show love, he will surely at the same moment kill the patient' (ibid.: 195). The intermingling of love and hate reactions in the analyst's countertransference reactions when working with psychotic patients, suggest for Winnicott, that in the patient's early life there occurred 'an environmental failure at the time of the first object-finding instinctual impulses' (ibid.: 196).

Winnicott specifies the vast difference in early life between patients. Some patients who have had a satisfactory early experience are able to communicate this to the analyst unconsciously through the transference. Other patients, often those with psychosis, may have had deficient early experiences. The commencement of analysis may symbolise for such patients their first chance to experience and gain from the analyst a safe, secure environment. The provision of a stable environment is especially important in the analysis of patients with psychosis. For the neurotic patient, because they can formulate symbols, the environment of the analysis – such as the couch – can be taken symbolically as the warmth of the mother's love. As Klein and Bion suggest, a patient with psychosis finds difficulty in formulating symbols and will therefore think in concrete ways. The couch will literally stand for the analyst and their body, as Winnicott states: 'The couch *is* the analyst's lap or womb, and the warmth *is* the live warmth of the analyst's body' (ibid.: 199). This situation gives rise to a particular kind of emotional pressure on the analyst. According to Winnicott, analysts who work with psychotic patients are in a position that reflects that of a mother and her newborn baby. From the word go, he states, the mother hates her baby.

Winnicott offers a number of reasons why the mother hates her newborn baby. Some examples of these reasons include the danger posed by the baby (from its conception) to its mother's body, and the hurt done to the mother's body by suckling and biting. The baby also treats its mother like a slave and throws her away after getting what it wants; the baby is sometimes suspicious of its mother's food, making her doubt herself, the baby then feeds perfectly happily from anybody but its mother. To tolerate her hate for her baby, the mother has to tolerate it, without doing anything about it. A child needs hate to be able to tolerate the extent of its own hate. A sentimental environment does not enable hate to be sorted-out and tolerated. Therefore, according to Winnicott, it does not benefit the child. The analyst has to be like a devoted mother to their patient with psychosis. Unless the analyst can hate their patient, the patient will not be able to tolerate their hate of the analyst.

## Little: pitfalls and value of the countertransference

Margaret Little, in her paper, 'Counter-Transference and the Patient's Response to It' (1951), discusses countertransference reactions in the analyst that may potentially interfere with the analyst's capacity to interpret and understand the patient. For example, she warns that the analyst may unconsciously repeat the behaviour of the patient's parents and satisfy needs of their own rather than the needs of the patient. Little states that the countertransference reactions in the analyst involve their whole psyche, id, ego and super-ego and there is no clear differentiation between them. However, in terms of the analyst's work with patients with a psychosis, the id is primarily involved.

Following Klein's observations of the fragmented ego of an individual with a psychosis, Little states that the analyst inevitably identifies with the patient's id, due to limited access to the fragmented ego. This identification will be one that is narcissistic, she states, 'on the level of the primary love-hate' (1951: 36). The analyst's encounter with a person with a severely disintegrated personality has distressing implications for the analyst. Danger spots that are 'deeply repressed and carefully defended' (ibid.) are activated, as well as primitive defence mechanisms. However, Little states that this brings about potential for satisfactory therapeutic results. In the midst of this, a fragment of the patient's ego can identify with the analyst's ego bringing about the patient's capacity for object love. This process is achieved when the patient recognises that the analyst understands his fears and he can then take in or introject the therapist's ego as a good object. Through the analyst's contact with reality the patient can find his or her own sense of reality. Although this contact is precarious at first, the patient continuing to introject the external world through contact with the analyst can strengthen the patient's ego. The patient will also be able to invest in the external world with libido originally derived from the therapist.

Little specifies that the patient with a psychosis may not be able to form a transference because of their disintegrated personality and so the analyst necessarily has to identify with the patient's id. Consequently, the analyst's countertransference feelings are experienced as intense and disturbed. The experience of identifying with the patient's id due to their disintegrated ego may also be encountered by mental health staff other than analysts, in their everyday work with patients with a psychosis. Primitive defence mechanisms that are brought into play can be an intense experience for staff and it might be that talking through the mechanisms involved alleviates this intensity. Although this intensity causes anxiety, it is also the root to understanding and helping the patient. These processes are not fully acknowledged in mainstream mental health practice. There seems to be no clear articulation of the often-difficult countertransference reactions encountered by staff working with patients with a psychosis, and no attempt to better understand them in terms of the patient's lived experiences.

## Rosenfeld: transference and schizophrenia

Herbert Rosenfeld treated schizophrenic patients using psychoanalytic techniques. In his paper, 'Transference-Phenomena and Transference-Analysis in an Acute Catatonic Schizophrenic Patient' (1952b), Rosenfeld suggests a challenge to the view that psychotic patients cannot transfer as expressed by Freud. Rosenfeld suggests that there is not a lack of transference but, rather, a problem encountered in the recognition and interpretation of transference in schizophrenia. Unlike Winnicott and Little, Rosenfeld's emphasis is not on the countertransference, but on the transference in psychosis. Freud specified that in psychosis, there is a regression to the auto-erotic and/or narcissistic stage in development whereby the infant takes itself as its love object. The individual with a psychosis, therefore, does not appear to recognise an external object. Rosenfeld states that when someone with psychosis approaches an object either in love or hate, they become merged with it. That person will encounter phantasies and impulses to get inside the object in order to control it. Here Rosenfeld draws upon Klein's concept of projective identification. He states that the person with a psychosis cannot differentiate between 'me' and 'not me'.

Rosenfeld states that the placing of oneself into an external object signifies an early stage of development where object relations begin. He states: 'In my opinion the schizophrenic has never completely outgrown the earliest phase of development ... and in the acute schizophrenic state he regresses to this early level' (1952b: 458). Rosenfeld states that parts of the self placed into external objects become persecutory. In addition, the characteristic withdrawal of interest in the outside world is, according to Rosenfeld, due to the individual attempting to defend against persecutors from the external world.

Rosenfeld offers a clinical example of a schizophrenic patient whom he treated psychoanalytically. He saw this patient for an hour and a half every day except Sundays. Rosenfeld gives a detailed account of the way in which this patient transferred onto him repetitions of his early object relations. I will only give a few examples of this transference and Rosenfeld's response to it here. The patient states: 'I should have stayed longer!' According to Rosenfeld, this statement reveals that the patient had a wish for his father to stay longer in a certain situation. As a result of projective identification the patient had lost himself and merged with his father. Having been previously unsuccessfully treated by a 'Dr A', the patient fears repetition of this by stating: 'The Russians *were* our allies.' Dr A had been an ally but had turned against him, and the patient feared Rosenfeld would do the same. He asks Rosenfeld if he is Jesus, indicating the wish for Rosenfeld to perform miracles and make him well. The patient said Dr A had committed suicide and confused him with Rosenfeld, fearing he would do the same.

This patient feared, according to Rosenfeld, that when he placed himself in others, he could not get out again. Rosenfeld states with reference to this patient how the process of projective identification brings about the symptoms of the patient's schizophrenia:

> The patient shows signs of an object-relation, in which he has impulses and phantasies of forcing himself or parts of himself inside the object, which leads to states of confusion, to splitting of the self, to a loss of the self and to states of persecution in which visual and auditory hallucinations are pronounced.
>
> (ibid.: 463)

Rosenfeld states that consideration given to this process enables an understanding of transference phenomena in schizophrenic patients. In the analytic relationship there has to be an attempt by the analyst to enable the patient to take back parts of their fragmented self in order to restore and integrate the ego.

Rosenfeld describes how this patient transferred his feelings onto a part of his body, namely his bent finger. Referring to his finger the patient stated, 'I can't do any more, I can't do it at all'. He proceeded to point to Rosenfeld's finger and said he was afraid of it. Initially his own finger had symbolised his feelings of depression. However, feeling that he could not cope with these feelings, he then projected them onto the finger belonging to Rosenfeld.

The process whereby the patient with a psychosis merges with others is described by Rosenfeld as being due to their inability to differentiate between 'me' and 'not me'. This indicates for staff involved in a psychotic patient's care, that they may consciously or unconsciously perceive a patient as psychically *getting inside* them. I describe this feeling in my observations of patients in Chapter 8. This may explain the often-expressed anxiety by staff working with such patients. However, if these counter-transference feelings were acknowledged, then this would be beneficial to staff in their work with patients, and they would be able to better articulate the meanings behind patients' verbal and non-verbal expressions.

In another paper, 'Notes on the Psycho-Analysis of the Super-Ego Conflict in an Acute Catatonic Patient' (1952a), Rosenfeld states the importance of the analyst using their countertransference reactions as a 'kind of sensitive "receiving set"' (1952a: 116). According to Rosenfeld, the analyst, through their countertransference responses, can form a better understanding of patients with a psychosis, especially as these patients often have great verbal difficulties. He states that such patients are often unable to use symbols. With neurotic patients, they take words from the analyst symbolically. In the case of psychotic patients, they take the words very concretely. Rosenfeld states that if the analyst interprets something the patient says as a castration phantasy, for example, the patient will actu- ally take the interpretation itself as a castration. Therefore, the analyst has to carefully convey their understanding of the patient they have gained from their countertransference reactions. They also have to observe the patient's verbal and non-verbal responses.

## Bion on containment in the countertransference

In his paper, 'Attacks on Linking' (in Bion 1993), Bion gives an example of an analytic situation echoing an early scene between a patient and their mother. In a clinical example, Bion describes a patient of his who expresses frequent displays of unprovoked aggression. This patient frequently attempts to rid himself of his fear of death and dying. He experiences these as too powerful and he attempts to split them off and projects them into the figure of Bion, his analyst. According to Bion, the patient felt that if his violent feelings could remain within his analyst for long enough they would undergo change and then be safely taken back inside. However, the patient felt that Bion had destroyed these feelings and they had become even more painful. Consequently, the patient forced his feelings into Bion in a more violent and persistent way, becoming more frightened as he carried out this process. Bion considers this to be a violent response to what the patient perceived as Bion's hostile defensiveness.

The patient, according to Bion, appears to be describing an early experience whereby his mother responded to his demands in a dutiful way. Bion couldn't help hearing on the part of the mother, a desperate, impatient, 'I don't know what's the matter with the child' (1993: 104). According to Bion, the mother needs to have acknowledged that the child required more than a demand of her physical presence. Bion states that this particular patient clearly had a mother who could not tolerate her child's feelings and demands. She either denied them altogether or took in – or introjected – her child's bad feelings. Bion states that the mother needs to feel and experience the child's disturbance herself. Bion states: 'From the infant's point of view she should have taken into her, and thus experienced, the fear that the child was dying. It was this fear that the child could not contain' (ibid.). Bion states that through the process of analysis, the analyst has to be able to contain the demands of the patient, just as the mother may be able to 'contain' feelings that her child has projected onto her. Furthermore, Bion points out that the mother is able to experience these feelings and contain them, and still 'retain a balanced outlook' (ibid.). In his paper, 'A Theory of Thinking' (in Bion 1993), Bion continues to discuss this theme. He states how the mother can take her infant's fear of death inside herself and at best tolerate them. The mother can then respond therapeutically and make the infant feel it can take back its fear in a form it can tolerate. Bion states the mother does this by her capacity for reverie. She therefore turns the baby's feelings into alpha elements and thus into conscious awareness and thinking. Thus, the mother has turned a thing-like or bodily experience, into a thinkable idea that is tolerable. Bion suggests that the analyst can also achieve this within the analytic situation.

## Searles: the analyst's unconscious

Harold Searles was another theorist who treated schizophrenic patients using intensive psychoanalytic psychotherapy. In his paper, 'The Schizophrenic's Vulnerability to the Therapist's Unconscious Processes' (1964), Searles states that schizophrenic patients not only project or transfer unconscious material onto the analyst, but also introject the unconscious processes of the analyst. Such patients will take on aspects of these unconscious processes, making them part of their own personality. Searles describes one particular patient who picked up his posture, awkwardness and views he temporarily had of himself as unkempt. The patient stated about herself: 'I know I'm a slovenly person.' Searles states in response: 'The frightening thing was that she evidently genuinely experienced these traits as being aspects of herself and was quite unable to perceive them as traits of mine' (1964: 198). Searles states this process stems from an individual's early experience of object relations. He considers that the infant, to try to relieve anxiety in its parents, introjects this anxiety inside of itself.

Searles describes how another patient of his was prone to outbursts of aggression, belches, flatus, dropping cigarette ash onto the rug and picking his nose. This patient also heard voices that were taunting and contemptuous that he would talk back to. Searles describes his realisation that the patient's voices were, in fact, echoes of himself that were introjected by the patient. The patient had introjected Searles' unrealised contempt for him. Thinking that he had just perceived this patient as desperate and suffering, Searles realised his contempt: 'My thought was "There goes that son of a bitch!" accompanied by a most intense feeling of contempt towards him' (ibid.: 202). As Searles realised his contempt for this patient and understood it as a countertransference response, and conveyed it to the patient, the hallucinations ceased.

According to Searles, analysts must possess a healthy ego so they can be sure of their perceptions of others. In this respect the analyst will not need confirmation from others that he perceives in a realistic way. Searles also states the importance of the analyst realising what psychic material belongs to him and what belongs to patients. Analysts also have to be able to acknowledge their often-disturbing countertransference reactions. According to Searles, the psychotic patient's ego is too weak to be secure in its perceptions of others. If the patient perceives that the analyst feels murderous towards him and the analyst does not relate this to him, the patient is likely to experience a hallucination of a murderous threat. Searles states that this is because the analyst has not acknowledged his/her countertransference reactions: 'We may say, the therapist has refused to accept the perception as being truly applicable to himself as "belonging here upon me"' (ibid.: 207).

Searles considers that intense transference on the part of the patient will produce feelings that are just as intense in the therapist. He suggests that the therapist will not merely stand for a parental figure in the transference process, such as in the case of neurotic transference. To the patient with a psychosis, the therapist will actually become like the parental figure, and the patient will manipulate the relationship in order for this to occur. Searles states that as well as behaving like the patient's parent, the therapist will actually experience painfully intense feelings that were present in the patient's childhood. Through the process of projection and introjection in the relationship he has with the patient, the therapist will experience 'the comparably intense and conflictual emotions which formed the seed-bed of psychosis in the child himself, years ago' (1964: 522).

It is vital that hatred is acknowledged between the therapist and patient so as to enable the hate to be bearable. This provides a basis for the next stage of love and commitment, before love and hate are integrated.

Referring to the treatment of schizophrenic patients in a hospital setting, Searles considers that hatred felt by the therapist is often repressed and projected onto various authoritative figures within the hospital, rather than being acknowledged. Having outlined the concept of psychical counter-transference as indicating the feelings evoked in the analyst that inform them about the patient's unconscious, I shall now turn to the work of Susie Orbach who describes this process at a bodily level.

## Orbach on body countertransference

Although there has been an increasing amount of literature on psycho-analytic theory and the body, the psychoanalytic writer Susie Orbach dis-cusses countertransference as experienced physically. In *The Impossibility of Sex* (1999), she describes her bodily reactions to her patients experi-enced during her work as a psychotherapist, which she terms as 'body countertransference'. This differs from conventional psychoanalytic theory, which focuses upon countertransference at a psychical level.

Orbach presents hypothetical encounters with patients who represent aspects of the phenomena of transference and body countertransference. She gives as one example of this, the case study of 'Edgar'. She describes how she feels she is growing bigger in response to him entering the consulting room. Orbach's responses turn out to be symbolic of Edgar's feelings, which he had been unable to recognise concerning his grand-mother's physical presence that he valued, and her subsequent departure. Orbach states: 'he had been trying to communicate something about her through his corporeal invocation of her in me. I needed to think about how to use what had been physically elicited in me' (1999: 112). Just as the theorists above describe how psychical feelings that arise in the analyst in response to the patient, as a result of the rapport between them, can be made use of as an effective analytical tool, Orbach describes this at a phys-ical level. Edgar's feelings about his grandmother – her valued physical presence and physical movement away from him – had emerged within the body of the analyst. Consequently, the analyst can strive to make sense of their bodily reactions in order to make sense of the patients' sense of their own and others' corporeality.

Orbach formulates body countertransference in three ways. First, the therapist may encounter a physical experience that has been absent in the development of the patient. Orbach gives an example of a patient who had hated her body and had never felt she had belonged within it. Orbach, while encountering this patient, experienced an overwhelming contentment with her own body. This offered her the opportunity to help her convey to the patient her wish for secure bodily boundaries, which the patient had evoked in her. This enabled the patient to make sense of and begin to leave behind her feelings of hating her own body.

The therapist in his/her direct encounter with the patient's body can also experience body countertransference. This encounter enables the patient's physical distress to enter the relationship. Orbach gives the example of a female patient who routinely pulled up her chair in order to sit extremely close to her therapist who, in turn, felt physically invaded by this gesture. Orbach and her patient came to understand this action as symbolic of the patient's own physical development in which she frequently vomited and bed-wetted, and the unstable feelings about her physicality which she appeared not to understand in terms of her body's beginning or end. Orbach states: 'my experience that she was pushy, that she evoked in me a desire to move back from her, was a hint about her possible body instability and her anxiety about physical connection' (ibid.: 207).

Orbach describes the third formulation of body countertransference as the therapist experiencing the physical state of the patient. She gives the example of a patient's fatigue that can then be felt by the therapist allowing insight into the patient's bodily state. Orbach thus argues that as well as paying attention to psychic countertransference feelings as theorised in traditional psychoanalytic theory, bodily countertransference can provide a wider insight into the physical development of the individual, which she considers as equally important to emotional development. The therapist's bodily countertransference helps the therapist understand something of the patient's lived experience, and thereby can begin to feed it back in terms of experience rather than body or thing-like symptom.

An emphasis upon body countertransference indicates that in a thera-peutic setting, therapists may experience bodily sensations that inform them about the physical development of the patient and their perceptions about their own and others' corporeality. I would contend that it is not easy to distinguish between physical and psychical responses to the patient and the two often intermingle. The feeling of disgust for example, can be experi-enced both psychically and physically. The psychical response whether innate or culturally learned, brings about a sense of aversion. The physi-cal experience is a tight feeling in the stomach, a wish to flee or a feeling of nausea. When experiencing a sense of disgust towards someone who hasn't washed for a prolonged length of time, for example, it is difficult to distinguish between what is felt physically and what is felt psychically. Here we can say that countertransference and body countertransference appear to overlap.

## Applying countertransference to clinical practice: some problems

The analytic situation enables the patient to unconsciously transfer or project unresolved, repressed conflict onto the analyst. The countertrans-ference or body countertransference experiences that are evoked in the analyst serve to give clues to these unconscious conflicts that have arisen and been repressed during the course of patients' psychical or physical development and their current psychological situation. A question arises as to whether such conflicts are always unconsciously transferred onto the analyst, or whether they are transferred due to a conscious intent.

In traditional psychoanalytic theory, Freud proposed that the analyst must go through personal analysis to strive to overcome their counter-transference feelings. Subsequent to Freud, theorists advocate that personal analysis enables analysts to have access to their own unconscious so as to distinguish between the feelings that belong to them and those that belong to the patient. In addition, it is important to acknowledge that many of the psychical and physical responses evoked in the analyst – including disgust, tiredness and so forth – may be an indication of the analyst's wish to detach or protect themselves from the feelings evoked in them by the patient. The responses I describe in my accounts of patients in Chapter 8, such as coldness or tiredness, may be an indication of the lived experiences of these patients, as well as my wish to detach or disassociate myself.

I propose that the concepts of countertransference and body counter-transference need to be incorporated into clinical practice. If clinical staff are aware of these concepts and can acknowledge their own counter-transference feelings, they may be more open to what patients' bodily presentations signify in terms of their lived experience. Do I then go as far as suggesting that clinical staff must also undergo personal analysis in order, as the theorists above suggest, to have access to their unconscious and therefore gain a more open and insightful approach to the transferred feelings of the patient? Or is acknowledgement and awareness on the part of staff to their countertransference feelings enough for them to be able to more effectively gain insight into the patient. Also, how would staff be made aware of these concepts and how would they be incorporated into clinical practice? Furthermore, how would staff work effectively with the knowledge they have gained about themselves and patients from the acknowledgement of their countertransference feelings? I shall raise these questions and attempt to provide answers to them in the concluding part of this book in Chapter 9.

## Conclusion

In this chapter I have discussed Freud's views about transference and countertransference in relation to neurosis and psychosis. He considers that patients with psychosis find it difficult to form a transference onto their analyst. In contrast to this view, I outlined the writings of Winnicott, Little, Bion, Rosenfeld and Searles who each consider that a patient with a psychotic illness transfers or projects unconscious material onto the therapist who, in turn, experiences countertransference responses that are often intense and painful.

Each acknowledges the difficulty of working with such patients and states the importance of the therapist having undergone their own analysis and acknowledging their own emotions in response to their patients. Orbach stresses the importance of acknowledging bodily responses to patients in psychoanalytic treatment, which may indicate clues to the patient's physical development and current psychological situation. These theories emphasise that reactions in the analyst are a vital aspect of the therapeutic relationship. They also focus on how the analyst, through attention to their own countertransference responses, can feed back the patient's thing-like or bodily symptoms as experiences or thinkable ideas (I will discuss this issue in Chapter 9).

The treatment of psychotic patients using intense psychoanalytic psychotherapy has largely fallen into disrepute. Large numbers of patients with a psychotic illness are treated with anti-psychotic medications, and are often offered practical help such as 'social-skills' training and occupational therapy. However, I consider that the ideas expressed by the theorists above are beneficial in the treatment of patients. I consider that mental health professionals, other than therapists, encounter countertransference reactions in their everyday encounters with psychotic patients.

The recognition of countertransference and the difficult psychical and physical responses it stirs up in staff is not articulated within mainstream psychiatry. There is little encouragement for staff to attempt to examine their psychical and physical reactions in order to understand themselves and their patients better. The theorists I have outlined all specify the importance of this. If such ideas were applied to clinical practice, and staff could be helped to recognise their countertransference reactions, they might be better placed to understand their patients' lived experiences. These ideas also serve to individualise patients rather than placing them into universal diagnostic categories. This would also serve to create an intelligent working environment where reflective clinical practice would be encouraged as well as a format for the discussion of staff reactions.

In the next chapter, I present four case studies of patients diagnosed with mental illness. I provide a brief biographical background to each person and describe my observations and interviews with them. I offer my interpretations of what they might be communicating through their bodily presentation. I also include attention to transference and countertransference – plus body countertransference – issues.

# Chapter 8

# The patient's body

In this chapter, I present my accounts of the four patients I observed and interviewed at a day hospital. I provide a brief biographical background to each. These details came mostly from the accounts of their lives the patients generously gave me (the patients and their psychiatrists, as well as the staff team, also gave me permission to read the patients' notes if required). I provide my interpretations of the meanings apparent in their bodily presentation. I also describe my responses to the patients during the process of our interactions. As I have stated, I consider it is useful for staff to pay attention to, and make sense of, their reactions and responses in order to understand their patients better.

This approach of paying attention to our responses to the people we care for rather goes against a popular technique used by researchers referred to as 'bracketing', whereby the researcher puts aside their emotional responses and assumptions. This process is thought to enable the researcher to listen more fully to the person they are interviewing (Nieswiadomy 1998). As I discussed in the previous chapter, responses such as tiredness, fear and anger may reflect unconscious intentions on the part of the patient. Also, I consider that these responses may be fed back to the patient to help them make sense of, and further communicate, their distress. Therefore, I did not want to put my values and feelings aside when observing and inter- viewing the patients, as 'bracketing' suggests.

The day hospital was intended for people who lived in the community, but was also attended by patients who were in-patients in some of the adjoining wards. The day hospital had a warm atmosphere and offered a range of activities (including a gym) such as relaxation and discussion groups, a women's group and various art therapies. I worked closely with the staff team during my time there, and they were very welcoming. We devised a plan of action in the event of any distress occurring to the patients as a result of the interviews. Of course, some of the patients did become upset during the interviews, but I ensured that I interacted closely with the staff team so that additional support could be given if needed.

As I stated earlier, I left some leaflets about my research at the day hospital for patients to respond to. Many of the patients approached me to ask questions to find out more about the research. From the start, I noticed differences between the men and women in this process. I had observed from my first day at the day hospital that the men and women used the space in very different ways. The men appeared to take up more space and seemed to have a more assured physical presence. The women, however, formed a small group in the seating area and appeared to be more reticent about taking up space. In terms of my research, the men volunteered readily. As I state below, Turan was hesitant about the interview because he wondered if his life would be complicated for me. But overall I was aware the men felt *important* enough to participate.

The women were much more hesitant. The women spoke about their bodies very much in terms of the outside. It was as if they were considering their physical appearance and attractiveness from the perspective of someone else. That external gaze, it seemed, was deprecating and critical. I explained to all patients who asked me about the research, that I was interested in asking people about their feelings and experiences of their bodies and that I wanted to observe them. The men seemed to accept this quite happily. The women, however, seemed worried that I was going to judge or criticise their bodies. Perhaps consequently, they brought my body into our interactions. Their message was quite clear – I was visible and had stature in comparison to them. I felt that this related to my status (perhaps as a 'sane' woman, asking all the questions?) rather than to the fact that I'm almost six feet tall. The women seemed to suggest that they were rather unimportant, and did I really want to bother about them?

In various ways, the people I present below each experienced an incomplete or fragile sense of self. What is important to note here is that our relationships with others depend, as Murray Jackson states, on our capacity to distinguish ourselves from other people (2001: 176). In psychosis, as we have seen, the sense of self is often fragmented. The person experiences, literally, 'bits' of themselves in other people and objects. As the case study of Turan suggests below, he experienced parts of himself and other people in a variety of concrete objects. The perspectives I outline in this book suggest that the formation of a complete and assured sense of self is very much related to the infant's early experiences. Freud and Schilder, for example, argue that an infant gains its sense of self – its ego – from early bodily sensations arising on the surface of its body, the libidinal investment of bodily zones, and its interaction with its primary caregiver. These interactions involve the early experiences and negotiations of being fed, toileted and so forth. The baby internalises the hopes and fears of its primary caregiver. Whether or not this process was straightforward for the people below, it is absolutely clear from their accounts, that their life experiences – including their early experiences – had often been disruptive, stressful and traumatic. Perhaps these experiences had contributed to their mental distress.

These perspectives tend to, perhaps unfairly, blame the parents, particularly the mother. Parents, of course, do their best in the psychological, physical and social circumstances they are in. However, it does appear that a person's early experience does seem to influence their transition to adulthood. This point constitutes the main focus of the psychoanalytic profession. Other professions often vehemently deny this and argue that the here and now is surely important. Yet, I wonder if it is possible to just detach our pasts from ourselves. I can say that most of the people I have worked with in my capacity as mental health practitioner have had disruptive, fragmented and often distressing experiences. On the other hand, perhaps we could say, haven't we all? Is it just that some of us cope better than others?

As stated, in the case studies that follow, I offer my interpretations of the meanings apparent in patients' bodily presentations using aspects of the perspectives outlined in this book. I frequently ask questions about these possible meanings. I suggest that various 'symptoms' do often have meaning. However, I do not claim to have definitive answers to everything. I am not a trained psychoanalytic psychotherapist. I have, however, had my own personal psychoanalysis lasting several years. That has not made me some kind of ideal, perfect or special person or practitioner. However, I feel that analysis has sensitised me towards dynamics in personal and professional relationships (but, of course, one does not get it right all of the time). Whether or not it is useful or necessary for all nurses to undergo therapy in order to work effectively with patients, I nevertheless feel that awareness of oneself is crucial in work with disturbed people. I discuss this issue further in the concluding chapter.

I found being with the patients mentioned in the following interviews very difficult at times, but I felt I wanted to listen to what they had to say. I think it is crucial for practitioners to be able to bear the distress of their patients. Through the ability to stay with patients and through attending to the responses we encounter in relation to them, we may gain some insight into how that person perceives and relates to the world. This is not easy and the practitioner will experience a range of 'negative' (as well as positive) feelings and responses, including tiredness, fragmentation, suffocation and even hatred. As we have seen from the perspectives I outlined in Chapter 7, these responses are very understandable and human. They are also useful in the understanding of our patients. I consider that attention to symptoms and the meanings apparent in them and the effects they have upon us, allow us to spend time with our patients and listen to what they are saying. Consequently, this process enables us to understand them better and, crucially, to consider their mental illness in the context of their life experiences. In this way we may become respectful practitioners. What follows, of course, is the question of how our insights might help our patients. I will discuss this more fully in the next chapter. I wish to point out that the reader might find these accounts rather fragmented in themselves. I wanted to present them as they occurred. I did not want to save all my interpretations to the end. These are situated, or rather scattered, within my accounts of my interactions with the patients, along with my reactions and responses.

## Turan

My interactions with Turan took place during one interview and then for several weeks at the day hospital while I was conducting other interviews. Turan, who was forty-five years old, attended the day hospital while he was an in-patient on a ward. He had been sectioned under Section 3 of the Mental Health Act. He was Turkish-Cypriot and had lived in England since 1969. He had grown up in Cyprus. He described it as a beautiful place, but he could not remember much of it. He expressed that he was unsure of who he was, nobody had told him: 'I'm not sure of my age', he said, 'I haven't been told the real facts'.

He initially declined taking part in the interview, 'I might be too complicated for you', he stated, and proceeded to suggest other patients in the day hospital who might have been good candidates. Turan talked at length about the importance of gaining information and facts about things. He then approached me again and stated he was keen to take part. He explained he had endured some terrible physical injuries as a child that were, to him, 'very significant'. Again, he warned me that he might be complicated for the purposes of my research.

Turan was very charming and polite. He was tall and thin and often wore very colourful shirts that were bright and dazzling. He walked in a controlled, stiff way leaning towards the right hand side of his body. I observed that Turan clutched this side of himself as if, I thought, he was trying to hold himself together, or rather to hold two halves of himself together. Turan's face had lots of expression. His face was very mobile and he frequently moved his eyebrows and the corners of his mouth. He repeatedly blinked and flashed his eyes. He also often looked suspicious and guarded. He talked to me at some length about the differences in what we could both observe around us. 'You can see people behind me, but I cannot see what is behind me. I know there are lots of people lurking about.' When he sat down with his legs folded, the top leg began to swing, almost violently, backwards and forwards. I observed that these leg movements were probably due to medication. Turan was prescribed an anti-psychotic medication named Olanzapine.

In his notes, Turan was presented as suffering from paranoid schizophrenia and experiencing thought disorder and paranoia. It was also noted that Turan was described as experiencing the negative symptoms of schizophrenia. These were described in bodily terms. They included inability to attend to self-care and poor sleep and appetite. Turan was unable to manage when he was unwell. He became cut off and isolated and did not manage to pay his bills so they all piled up. The professionals caring for him then went through the process of contacting British Gas and so forth, informing them that Turan had been unwell.

Turan first came into contact with the psychiatric services in 1980. He referred to himself as a 'revolving door patient'. I read in his notes that while in hospital, he often discharged himself before he was well enough to go home. Consequently, on this particular admission he was sectioned. In addition, his father had died a year ago, so it was thought that he needed more support. In his notes, it was stated that Turan's mother lived near him, but she wanted him to stop visiting her. He often accused her of cursing him and she found this frightening and upsetting. Turan expressed this curse upon him to me. 'She curses me day and night, it's happening all over the place, I cannot break the curse', he stated. Throughout our many conversations, it seemed that Turan's parents, or the effect they seemed to have upon him, were symbolised in the many delusions and hallucinations he expressed.

On the evening before the interview with Turan, I had eaten lots of garlic (baked in their skins). At the time of the interview, Turan noticed this, and commented, 'Have you been eating garlics this morning?' He stated that the smell was rather warm and appealing. But more specifically, garlic would protect me, he suggested. It would protect me from the snake. He proceeded to tell me a story about a snake. There were a lot of snakes around where he grew up in Cyprus, as well as rather beautiful chameleons and lizards. He stated that if you are lost in the desert and wished to sleep, you could lie down and surround yourself with garlic. 'Then the snake won't get you', he said. The issue of the snake re-emerged frequently during our conservations: 'The slivery snake is dangerous', he told me, 'it doesn't know where it's going, it's out of control, it hisses at people, it is evil'. Later Turan said the snake was in his body and it was dead. What did this snake symbolise? The snake was, perhaps, a concrete representation of Turan's feelings about himself and others. If Turan was the snake, was he implying that I needed protection from him?

I asked Turan to tell me about his background. His speech was very disjointed and I felt muddled, disorientated and thrown off course. The disarray and muddle meant that the interview was tiring. Perhaps this was a reaction stirred up in me by how Turan experienced the world. I wondered if this is what he was trying to say when he warned me about being so complicated. I started to feel, as Little and Rosenfeld have stated in their observations of interacting with psychotic people, that his words got into me. They didn't quite feel like words. They seemed rather deadening and intrusive, although Turan himself was very lively.

Rosenfeld suggested that the person with psychosis often cannot distinguish between 'me' and 'not-me', and frequently experiences a merging with other people or things. Although Turan was extremely likeable, I still felt rather intruded upon and suffocated. I felt I couldn't keep up with him and that he really was disjointed and fragmented. As I stated above, I felt that the complication Turan had warned me about was, in fact, his feeling of fragmentation. Consequently, I had a strong desire to bring everything together, for his benefit and mine.

Turan said that as a child, while growing up in Cyprus, he had been tormented. He had grown up in a secular Islamic environment. My observation of his body appearing to be experienced by him in two halves or broken in some way, began to make more sense when he spoke about an early operation he had. This was, in fact, a delusion. He stated that he had an operation and his leg was amputated (although it clearly had not been, I saw the skin on both of his feet in the sandals he wore). His leg was open, he said, and they took him to another place and they stitched it back together again. Turan described how he was disabled on his right side. As stated, I certainly observed how he held on to this side of his body while he walked. 'I have injuries from my toe to my heart', he said. Below his knee, he said, he had had a radioactive metal plate inserted. He told me how doctors had looked at his right side with a nuclear scan and there was an infection in the bone of his leg. Turan stated how he had rubbed a hole in his leg with a wet cloth and the infection was freed. He said the leg still remains with some infection in it – 'like a dead snake', he exclaimed, he had killed the snake, 'the snake is dead'. At this point he rolled up his trouser leg to show me the open infected wound, which I could not see. I was moved by the noises he made to indicate how much it hurt him. He explained that as a consequence of his injuries he could not pray.

Turan described these injuries as representing his 'feministic side'. I asked him to say a bit more about this. He replied that he believed that God is a woman. 'Yet femininity is strong', he said, 'it's to do with the way the body develops and education, it makes us strong'. This female god was, as he told me, in the good left hand side of his body. In the 'non-disease part', as he put it. It seemed to me that this good side represented his perceptions of the good parts of him. It also felt he wanted this side – like a good, comforting mother – to repair the injuries inherent in the bad and diseased parts of him. His mother had, in fact, cursed him. He experienced these curses in a range of different objects, as we shall soon see. It gradually came to the fore during the process of our interaction, that Turan had split himself in two – good and bad. These aspects were inside and outside of him, which he seemed to both communicate and experience in physical terms.

I asked Turan how old he was when this operation occurred and he replied that he didn't know. He stated that he didn't remember anything before primary school. Turan then said, however, that he remembered the operation. The doctors and nurses were saying that they'd had enough of him and that his parents were coming to take him home. He said, 'I didn't know who my mum and dad were, I thought they can be real and I should love them'. However, when they came to get him, which they must have done at some point to take him home, he couldn't recognise them. It then occurred to him that he could remember aspects of his life prior to primary school. He was five years old and his grandmother was lying on the floor in the doorway of her house. Turan said how he had jumped over her. He stated, 'A big curse was put on me to make me make mistakes'.

He returned to the subject of his parents. They had always cursed him, he said. They had told him he wasn't educated enough. It seemed that they were very strict and repeatedly told him to say his prayers. He stated that he needed to say his prayers, but he was not trained to pray. As a result, he felt he was not 'orthodox', or in other words, a strict Muslim like his parents. He returned to this issue several times during the course of the interview. He had not said his prayers and was not 'orthodox', he repeated. It seemed that this was the reason for his being cursed, not only by his parents, but also by the rest of the world.

Turan talked at length about being cursed. It was rather muddled, but he stated that people were always cursing him. There were people 'always lurking about and, coming up behind him', he said. They were always whispering and blaming him. Clasping his head, he spoke of 'bad things', 'cannabis, fighting, Satanism and sex, they don't help anything'. He then proceeded to describe his siblings. He had a sister who was very much like him, he said. Turan's brothers often beat her up. His three brothers were always, in Turan's words, 'pressing his weak points'. In comparison to his brother, Turan seemed to experience an unstable sense of manhood and felt weak. 'Many people would not like to know them', he stated. Turan described them as bad characters. One especially, he said, was a drug addict and alcoholic. This brother often attacked his mother, Turan said, 'on her elbow'.

Turan described his father as a proud man who had fought in the war. He was a member of the military police in Cyprus. Turan said his father was always boasting about his achievements and strength. Turan stated: 'He was strong, he didn't suffer.' With this comment, although he didn't say it, I heard Turan say, 'not like I did'. It seemed that the father was a frightening man. Turan described how he was once ill and in need of an ambulance. 'I couldn't breathe', he said, 'I was suffocating'. His father held Turan's hands behind his back to prevent him from getting help. Turan also described how he used to hide in the dark so his father would not see him. He also secretly read books that were 'non-Islamic'. Some of the UN British troops would give him books and money. 'I conversed with them', he said, 'and didn't tell anyone'. He described how for ten to fifteen years he had watched his father praying. It seemed to me that he was caught between the values inherent in his background and those symbolised by those outside, such as those espoused by the British troops. 'I myself was weak', Turan said. It seemed that he managed always to come through, as he put it, with the help of a good spirit. In contrast, there was also the presence of an evil spirit, which was also instrumental in cursing Turan and his life.

The 'Good Spirit', as Turan described it, was a guardian angel. 'Lady luck, a lease of life', he said. He described the 'Evil Spirit' as orthodox and bearded. Was this his father, or aspects of him? The Evil Spirit had tried to help Turan with problems in his childhood, but he had a real problem trying to survive, 'he was perspiring an awful lot'. Turan stated that the Evil Spirit would be submerged in water with his arms stretched out, trying to float. 'I find it hard to enter the spiritual world', he said, 'I'm not orthodox'. He described how his Evil Spirit had arranged for photographs to be taken of Turan. These photos came out in 1992, he said. They were taken to a court of law, he said, and were 'indicated by a judge'. According to Turan, it was revealed in court that Turan was 'shadowy', 'these photos were taken by entanglements', he stated. 'They were wiring me up. I feel so tense in my body, my Evil Spirit has been with me, sweating, he was suffering.' Turan described the Evil Spirit as himself, as if he were entangled. He described again how the Evil Spirit was sweating like hell, he said, 'so to indicate the difficulty I was facing'.

Turan then described his 'Good Spirit', which he referred to as having a male persona. 'He is perfection', Turan stated, 'like James Bond or Sean Connery, like a monk'. He then proceeded to inform me how the good spirit was changed. Turan was in his house and he smelt something burning, the police were trying to break through the window. Turan stated that he could sense something evil coming to capture him. 'They had to go through these things', he said, 'the prison guards, the judge, so many burdens'. He then described a small house martin, 'or a swift or a swallow'. This small bird seemed to represent himself as a vulnerable bird not able to fly away, in the middle of the floor. This bird was neither awake nor asleep. 'They keep pestering me', Turan stated, 'they won't leave me alone'. He said 'How many Turans are there in the world? How would they cope with the curses?' I got a sense that Turan *felt* in bits and pieces, and wondered how the many parts of him, or the unified, complete him, would be able cope with being him.

I proceeded to ask Turan some questions about his bodily experience. How did he feel about looking in the mirror? He replied that sometimes he experiences severe anxiety around mirrors. 'The reflection hurts you', he said. He complained that there were mirrors everywhere trying to humiliate him. He then described his position in relation to me. 'I look at you, you feel good, I feel good – I don't feel like that looking in the mirror.'

Being with me seemed positive then? Did *being with* other people somehow help him feel supported or held together? Did my reflection make his experience more bearable? It seemed that Turan was able to separate and distinguish himself from me. Yet being with him I had felt countertransferentially, so suffocated and intruded upon. I was also surprised by his ability to see himself as separate, as he had been suggesting by his comments that he had experienced himself as fragmented and projected out into external objects. Following this discussion about looking in the mirror, Turan added that he saw someone else in the mirror, 'the one who curses me', he stated.

I asked Turan how he expressed his feelings. He replied that it was difficult for him to pinpoint his problems. He wanted a 'living space', he said. At this point he held his head and shut his eyes. He explained that the staff on the ward were always asking him assessment questions. These were related to his illness, he said. He gave examples such as, 'What is your name? How long have you been here? He complained that they never asked him "Hello, would you like a cup of tea?"' 'They never approach me like that'. Turan stated that the media and the authorities were always disclosing bad information that was damaging. I felt he was referring to information about his own life or, more specifically, his guilt at not being orthodox in the way his father had been.

I asked Turan how his body made him happy or unhappy. He again described his injuries: 'I was in hospital, I don't know how I got there', he stated. 'People look down on me', he said, 'they feel superior to me'. His speech seemed centred upon issues around his orthodoxy. I wondered if Turan had a sense of his body. He was very mobile, clutching himself, gesticulating with his hands, swinging his legs and moving his facial features. As a final question, I asked Turan how he would like to be seen by the outside world. He replied that he wished to see the burdens forced upon him. 'Something that faces the world', he stated. He described that he'd like to be anonymous and to have a moustache (not a beard like his Evil Spirit).

From my observation of and interview with Turan, I considered the mechanism of projection that Freud and Klein described. It seemed that Turan experienced resistance to becoming a strict Muslim like his parents, and felt some considerable guilt about this. He seemed to feel guilty about not being good enough. He thus projected his painful guilt out onto external objects. As I have stated, his resistance and guilt was concretely represented in various objects. However, they returned in a persecutory form. These objects were in the form of the mirrors that hurt him and the people who whispered about him and cursed him. These objects, it seemed, were also split into good and bad as symbolised by the evil spirit and the good spirit, who each took on Turan's physical and psychical experiences. Turan thus experienced himself as fragmented and multiple.

I wondered what his operation and the injuries to the right hand side of his body signified. Were these aspects of himself, perhaps his failure to comply with his parents' expectations of him as a strict Muslim? He had explained that he couldn't pray because of these injuries. It occurred to me that his injuries that made his body appear stiff, meant that he couldn't kneel down to pray. Thus, I considered that his body symbolised a site of psychical conflict.

Turan had also described his injuries as the 'feministic' part of him. I wondered if this too symbolised resistance on his part. In contrast to the God of Islam, God to Turan was a woman and symbolised strength and education. Did the femininity also signify his vulnerable side? It seemed that he attempted to hold onto this vulnerable side of himself as he walked along. Did he also feel that this side, which was perhaps valuable to him, was destroyed by the strictness of his upbringing? Was the femininity his good mother in his fantasy that didn't (as he experienced in reality) curse him? Was she protective like the good spirit? I also considered his reference to the dead snake, manifested in his leg. I wondered if this symbolised the rigid atmosphere of his upbringing that he wished to resist. Islamic faith is a complete submission to God, and the believer surrenders unconditionally to the divine will. Perhaps in Turan's experience, he did not wish to surrender himself in this way and this was symbolised within his body as a site of resistance and autonomy.

## Tom

Tom, who was forty-nine years old, was well known to the staff at the day hospital and other mental health services. He had been an in-patient six times over a period of seven years through several suicide attempts. Tom said to me these attempts to kill himself were a cry for help. Although, according to Tom, people weren't much help. He stated that they were equal in his mind to 'a pile of shit'. They were useless, he said. His cat meant more to him than other humans. 'I cut myself off', he stated, 'I completely blank people'.

In terms of his bodily presentation, Tom was tall and stocky and walked in a stiff, clumsy way. What was most noticeable about him was the way he dragged his right leg along with him and clutched it when he sat down. 'I can't stand for long, I'll have to sit down', he said when I first spoke to him. He actually couldn't bend his right leg, so he spread it out in front of him when he sat down. Tom lent forward to clutch it as if trying to protect it. He approached me, expressing his keenness to take part in the interview. 'I want to talk about my leg', he said, 'it's ruined my life', again frantically clutching it.

I observed how although Tom was always well dressed, he also had a strong body odour. He took up a lot of space in the way he spread out his leg. He leant back and stretched out his arms onto the chairs either side of him. He was very eager to take part in the interview, which I instantly felt as suffocating and somewhat pushy. 'Let's do it now', he said. I explained I needed to contact his psychiatrist to get their approval and to give Tom some time to think about it. 'I won't need any time to think about it, and I'll be available anytime.'

In his notes, Tom was described as suffering from depression with psychotic features for which he was prescribed antidepressant and anti-psychotic medications. He was also prescribed sleeping tablets. The bodily effects of his depression were detailed in his notes. He was described as having a history of self-harm such as cutting his arms. He would often present himself to the emergency clinic with cuts on his arms and threatening to cut his wrists. He would subsequently be admitted to an in-patient ward. He was also described as neglecting his self-care by not washing. This was particularly apparent when he was very depressed. His sleep and appetite were also poor at these times and he had low energy levels. Tom had frequent out-patient appointments with his psychiatrist and attended the day hospital for day-to-day support.

When the interview began, Tom provided me with some details of his life. I felt rather overwhelmed by his physical presence; something about him seemed to be filling up the room, or rather the space between us. Despite his exclamations about people being like shit to him, he was very well mannered and I didn't feel frightened of him. Tom told me he had been a dispatch rider for twenty-six years until an accident in 1995 prevented him from working altogether. He stated he liked this job because he got smelly and dirty in the process. 'Roaring through the dirty streets', he said, 'I looked a real state at the end of the day'. I picked up that he experienced pleasure in this. This was confirmed when he said he always made a point of being dirty, of putting people off, as he put it. 'Tough shit,' he said, if he offends people (and I felt this included me), 'well that's their business'. Tom did his best to put people off him. As I have described, I felt rather overwhelmed by him and rather suffocated, but I didn't find him off-putting. He had rather unpleasant body odour (body odour generally does not bother me very much), and had a rather intrusive way of taking up space. When I thought about it, I was overcome by his need of others more than anything, which was in sharp contrast to his desire to turn people away from him. This began to make sense as he began to tell me about himself. I felt he really wanted me in some way to experience his suffering.

Tom expressed strongly that he wanted to be isolated. He didn't go out, and hated crowds: 'Fucking cinemas and theatres and shops, I hate them, I avoid them like the plague.' If he went to the cinema, he said, he became claustrophobic and had fits. Tom told me he was once in the art room at the day hospital and somebody shut the door, and there he was on the floor when he woke up. His body was covered in bruises. Tom explained he'd endured a fit and collapsed and nearly 'smashed himself up'. 'I feel frightened', he said, 'if I'm left in a room on my own'. Tom had removed the interior doors from his flat as soon as he moved in, so as not to feel shut in. These fears, it seemed, related to some of his early experiences.

Tom was an only child and his mother had him when she was in her late thirties. In those days, in the early 1950s, he said, a woman having a baby in her late thirties was considered old. It seemed, from what his grandmother told him, that his mother was delighted when she became pregnant, she'd been trying to conceive for so long and 'she was about to give up'. 'Frequently fucked by my father', he said, 'but nothing got through for a long time'. However, his father left his mother and him when he was three. Tom said he couldn't remember this. The following year Tom was involved in a horrific car crash. He and his mother were travelling to the West Country to visit his grandmother when they crashed into another car. His mother, who was driving, was killed instantly. Tom was thrown through the windscreen of the car and landed on the road. A coach travelling in the opposite direction, as Tom put it, 'smashed my body to bits'. He received hospital treatment for his injuries for the next six years. He was in a coma for the first six months and then spent the next two years 'living in an operating theatre'. He learnt to walk again using a metal frame.

While Tom told me these details, he started to cry. 'Nobody told me my mother was dead', he said. It seemed that he wasn't told for a further two years. 'Okay, I was in a coma for the first six months, but nobody told me where my mum was when I woke up.' His grandmother came to see him, but he longed to see his mother. 'I kept asking where she was', he said, 'but nobody said a thing about her'. Then one day, his grandmother told him, and Tom was convinced she felt that he was to blame for his mother's death.

He proceeded to tell me the next terrible event in his life. At the age of ten, Tom was eventually discharged from hospital after being, as he put it, 'put back together by doctors and surgeons'. He went to live with his grandmother who, in his view, couldn't cope with him. She was elderly by that time, he explained, and he was always difficult. 'I made life impossible for her, I was so difficult', he stated. He explained how he was always brimming over with energy. I got a sense of him almost trying to burst out of himself, as if detached from his damaged physical frame. Tom also got easily bored. Consequently, he used to tear apart a loaf of bread or other items of food, leaving them over the floor in the hall, or rip up letters. 'I wanted to get inside the washing machine', he said, 'and go round and round'.

Tom started 'proper school' and made a few friends. School was also difficult for him. He explained that he 'walked in a funny way' as a result of his injuries. 'My bones were all mended, but I was still stiff, and bending my joints was difficult.' Some of the boys at school would torment him for this and call him 'stiffy'. However, despite these torments, Tom thought that being tall meant he dealt with these remarks. He mentioned that I was tall at this point and suggested that I felt strong like him. He asked me when I first 'became' tall and I described how I had always been tall and, consequently, expected to be great at sports at school. Returning to his life, he explained that he was so glad to get out of hospital, that he wasn't too bothered by the remarks. He, too, was expected to be sporty and he managed to engage in some activities despite his injuries. Tom then described how he believed he would eventually be able to fully recover. However, these apparent positive feelings were short lived.

Tom told me how he was then sent to live with his godfather. This meant changing school, which was rather distressing 'starting all over again'. In actual fact, he didn't attend school that much. 'There were bad things going on at home', he said. His godfather, along with three other men systematically abused him for the next six years. These men, as Tom described it, would smack him and hit him with kitchen implements. They told him it was God's punishment because he had killed his mother. Tom stated how he had 'forgotten' his mother by then 'and they brought her back'.

It seemed that prior to this abuse, Tom had been fantasising about his eventual physical recovery. This was now shattered. Tom described how these men made him crawl on the ground, and he felt, 'like a pile of shit'. Tom described this abuse in a frantic tone, as if he was running a marathon. He became short of breath, wiping the sweat off his brow. I also felt this anxiety in my tummy and felt rather dizzy. I felt a sensation of wanting to escape and get out of the room. Due to my physical reactions, I asked Tom if he wanted to stop the interview, as it seemed he was very distressed. I realised this question was more for my benefit than his. However, he said he felt okay, and that it helped to talk. Tom proceeded to tell me he also endured sexual abuse from these men. One in particular, Tom stated, 'used to ask me to suck him off'. Tom stated that he felt that he was kept in a cage for ten years and the only relief was some visits to his aunt.

When he was sixteen, Tom told his aunt what had been happening to him. I asked if he had felt able to tell her before, but he replied he was 'too frightened'. At sixteen, he'd again managed to build up some fantasies of getting better. His aunt listened to him with some suspicion, he said, but appeared to believe him. Tom's godfather was arrested and put on trial, but 'they' believed him rather than Tom. The judge apparently accused Tom of being a liar. He then went to stay with his aunt. He was convinced that she was always suspicious of his story. I felt Tom was trying to pressure me to believe him. 'You do believe me don't you?' he insisted. In response to this, and I do not intend to be dispassionate, I wasn't particularly interested as to whether this account was true or not. Obviously, Tom was trying to communicate something about him. I felt overall that he was trying to communicate his feelings about the loss of his mother at such a young age. In words, he had told me he had forgotten this event, but was it that he was trying to conquer or overcome his feelings through his various actions.

After leaving school, Tom became a dispatch rider. This surprised me considering the horrific accident he had experienced at the age of four. In fact, it seemed that dangerously tearing through the roads at a great speed was pleasurable to him. He was always 'tempting fate', he said, 'taking risks, overtaking and riding too fast'. He told me he was much like the cartoon character the 'road-runner'. In 1980, Tom met a woman, interestingly, on a bus. They began a brief relationship. He really liked her, he said, 'but in another way she meant nothing to me'. He said he always knew he would lose her. They had no sexual relationship and eventually parted.

In 1995, Tom had another accident: 'A truck crushed into me and my right leg was smashed up'. At the hospital, the doctors had to insert plastic inside his leg, which he described as still digging into his skin from the inside. Although he didn't say it in words, I took this to mean that the original accident where he had lost his mother was still hurting. His body had taken on this pain. Tom attempted to roll up the trouser leg of his damaged leg to show me the damage. There were visible scars from a series of lacerations. I felt squeamish as if I was looking at an open wound. I also got a sense of how significant Tom's leg was to him. He clutched it almost lovingly. 'It hurts', he exclaimed, and then said angrily, 'the whole fucking thing is made of plastic, and I'd rather have it cut off'. He sat clutching his damaged leg for the remainder of the interview.

His confrontations with road traffic emerged again five years later. Tom was accused of jumping on top of a car bonnet. The car was stationary on a quiet road at the traffic lights. He had heard voices telling him to do it, he told me. Tom informed the driver of his status as a mentally ill patient and they did not press charges. I asked him why he had done this and he replied that it was a 'strong desire, I just had to do it, they were telling me I had to do it'. Tom explained that he often heard voices telling him he was evil. These were particularly strong at times of stress. In Kleinian terms, he had expelled his pain, but it was represented in the voices he heard. Roaring around the streets had somewhat reduced them, he suggested. I felt that in these circumstances he was trying to conquer his guilt about his mother, or to somehow come close to her and the original 'event'. Again, he brought up his encounter with vehicles by stating he really wanted to return to work. He wanted to learn how to drive a bus so that he would be able to help his older neighbours in his estate with their shopping. He could collect them from the shops, he said, 'and take them safely home'.

I then proceeded to ask Tom some further questions relating to his experience of his body. At this point, I felt worn out as if it had been me tearing around the streets. Tom replied that he felt there was no life in his body. 'My body is dead and there is no life in it', he stated. Despite telling me his painful experiences, Tom's speech was also rather lifeless and deadening. I felt that perhaps he tried to deaden his feelings so as not to experience the full impact of them. Although his speech was deadening, I nevertheless picked up a sense of desperation in him that made an impact upon me. I felt rather overwhelmed and exhausted. Had Tom projected what I perceived as his feeling of desperate need for others into me? Was it this that was wearing me out? As I have stated, I think he desperately needed other people, but as a defence did his best to put people off.

I asked Tom about how he felt about looking in the mirror. Tom stated that he hated looking in the mirror and said he didn't look at mirrors if he could help it. However, he said while he was a dispatch rider he used to catch sight of himself in the side mirror of the bike. This was good, he said, he liked this image of himself. He 'was a free man and in control'. I asked Tom how he expresses his feelings. He talked some more about his claustrophobia and experience of black outs when the door is closed on him. He stated that he 'feels no emotion at all'. Continuing to clutch his leg, he explained his life was worthless. 'I feel dead, I don't feel my life is worth any amount of shit.' Everything and everybody had ruined his life. People meant nothing to him, he said. He said he would have no trouble killing someone who offended him. There were so many injustices he said. As an example of this, he talked about people who steal. He stated how usually he didn't agree with 'Arabs and their regimes', but the shariah method of cutting off the hands of those who steal, was in Tom's mind a good idea.

How did his body make him happy or unhappy? He described how much he resented his leg and again stated his wish to have it cut off. He said he never got a penny for his injuries, 'no compensation at all'. He stated that his body made him unhappy because he could not work anymore. He managed to get Incapacity Benefit and Disability Living Allowance, but they were not adequate. He returned to the two accidents he had experienced. He described how nobody thought about what he was going through, and nobody believed that he had experienced abuse at the hands of his godfather. His godfather 'was very charismatic', he said, 'he got away Scot free'.

In my observations of, and interview with Tom, I considered his sense of his body image and how his psychical and physical processes interrelated. Schilder, drawing upon the ideas of Freud, stated that the body image is greatly altered with the onset of psychological and physical distress. Organic or physiological disorders are influential in affecting the body image. On the other hand, psychical investments in organs, such as in the case of hypochondria, also serve to alter or influence the body image. The person with hypochondria, for example, will overly invest a particular part of their body with libidinal energy. As a defence, they will attempt to isolate this body part and treat it as alien. Bearing these ideas in mind, I felt that Tom's damaged leg and his relationship to it, was indicative of these processes. Certainly his car crash at the age of four and the smashing up of his body significantly influenced how he experienced himself. It seemed as if his sense of himself was severely shattered, so his body and then his smashed up leg came to signify his smashed up psyche. I felt Tom had a desire to get rid of his leg, to detach it from the rest of him, yet it was also important to him and symbolised himself. He seemed to clutch it desperately during the interview and I felt that this was an attempt to hold himself together in order to stop himself from falling to pieces.

According to Freud and Schilder a person's ego comes into being as a result of their bodily sensations and their identification with those in the outside world. Therefore, there is a clear correlation between psychical and physical processes. In these terms, a fragmented sense of self is felt as a fragmented body or vice versa. In Tom's case, his fragmented body seemed to symbolise his fragmented sense of self, which he appeared in his bodily gestures to attempt to hold together.

For Lacan, the infant attempts to defend against its real experiences of bodily fragmentation by creating an imaginary anatomy of wholeness and integration. Tom was, perhaps, even more desperate to do this. His fear of fragmentation was confirmed in reality by his body being smashed up in the car crash. Consequently, he must have felt desperate to hold himself together. Although his leg was clearly painful, it nevertheless symbolised a part of him. In psychoanalytic terms, he couldn't get rid of his leg as it was invested with libido. It seemed that his identity was significantly caught up with traffic – the crash at four when he lost his mother; his job as dispatch rider and the risks involved in this choice of career; the only relationship he told me about being the meeting of a woman on a bus; the jumping on top of a car bonnet; and the wish to drive a bus in order to help his neighbours.

I wondered why Tom wanted to repeat and re-experience the danger of crashing on a road. As Freud suggests, people often have a 'compulsion to repeat' early traumatic experiences in order to attempt to deal with them. I felt Tom both wanted to recreate the crash to affirm his identity and then to make repairs. The reparation, perhaps, was indicated by his wish to drive his elderly neighbours safely home, to do good things. He described how he felt guilty for his mother's death and was subsequently sexually and physically abused for her death. Perhaps by looking after people he would repair the damage he thought he had done to her. Tom's wish to do good was in a sharp contrast to his view of people as shit and his wish to kill people. It seemed that he wished, as Laing suggests, to turn people into dead things or stone, in response to the fear he felt from others and his lack of being whole and integrated.

I felt Tom also intentionally attempted to distance himself from others by being smelly. It made me feel somewhat intruded on within my own body. It was, perhaps, his desire to fill the space as a whole being and put people off. This outer self was, perhaps, quite effective at protecting the more needy inner self. I was reminded of Laing's description of the person's creation of an outside in order to protect the inner self, or the 'shut-up self'. Tom's inner self contained, in my opinion, his need of others that perhaps overwhelmed him (and certainly overwhelmed me). Instead of feeling this need, he did his best to put people off and claimed they were just shit. It seemed that this was something he felt he could really master and control.

I have provided accounts of two male mental health patients I observed and interviewed at a day hospital. I consider that they clearly expressed aspects of their emotional need through their bodies. This was most apparent in terms of what I perceived to be their lack of integration and cohesiveness. Tom appeared to experience his body and sense of self as smashed up and fragmented and this was apparent in his bodily gestures and actions, I felt he was attempting to hold himself together. He kept returning to the accident that killed his mother and severely damaged his own body, and attempted to make reparation by once again returning to the road, but this time by wanting to drive his elderly neighbours safely home. Turan appeared to express his cultural, as well as his emotional, experience through his body. His creation of his operation and subsequent damage to the right hand side of his body, which he clutched as he walked along, perhaps symbolised an articulated resistance to his orthodox upbringing. The fragmentation of these patients was particularly striking and distressing. I often felt, in my interactions with these men, a need to hold myself together. I experienced the sensation of being thrown off balance by their lack of grounding particularly disturbing. I will return to this point in my concluding chapter where I explore how nurses might be able to deal with, and process, their experiences of interacting with people who experience fragmentation. I will now detail my observations of, and interactions with, two women patients.

As I stated in the last chapter, the women were reluctant to come forward and take part in the study. A few of the women asked about the study, expressed an interest, but proceeded to speak in self-deprecating ways. Some stated that they did not dress well, others that they hated looking in the mirror and felt bad about their bodies. I considered that I needed to employ different means to encourage them to take part and make them feel more comfortable. I considered the possibility of a women's group. As it turned out, the women actually made their own group within the day hospital seating area. It was then easier for me to talk to them about my research within this group. I also felt that within their group, they felt more comfortable to ask me about my research and to talk about their bodies.

Prior to this, I asked the staff for advice as to how I would encourage women to participate in my research. One of the female staff suggested I left some colourful leaflets around containing pictures of women sunbathing or looking in the mirror, and 'women's objects' such as lipsticks. I was reluctant to do this, as I was keen to talk to women about how they communicated inner distress through their bodies and not to just focus upon what they looked like from the outside. I thought in response to talking to this member of staff, that when women talk 'bodies' they tend to adopt popular discourses of femininity. In other words, they tend to speak of make-up, slimness, dieting and so forth. As I was about to find out, the women in my research also did this. I concluded that although these expressions are often irritating and deadening, they nevertheless could be understood as metaphors of how the women felt and therefore need to be listened to and made sense of.

## Moira

Moira, who was fifty-nine, had returned to the day hospital after being discharged. She had been admitted to one of the wards following an overdose and was encouraged to attend the day hospital to keep herself occupied. At the start of my interview, she said to me that this was not her first suicide attempt: 'This is one of several.' She said she was feeling very low and the day hospital was a good support for her. The other women in particular, she said, were very supportive. They had all experienced similar things to her. Moira told me that she couldn't think of any reason for her low moods, they seemed to 'just happen'. Moira said she had been depressed for eighteen years. 'I have been in and out of mental institutions.' Moira stated that although she wanted to take part in my research, she didn't like herself and her body, as she was 'fat and ugly'. Her responses seemed to suggest that she perceived her body as if from outside. She also seemed to suggest that I would be likely to be critical of her appearance.

In terms of her bodily presentation and appearance, Moira was indeed very heavy. She also had a strong body odour. Her hair was greasy and she appeared not to care about herself and her appearance. I found myself reacting to her appearance and smell. I heard many of the staff say that they wanted to tell Moira to have a bath. I also felt like this. However, I felt that Moira's bodily presentation might have had a significant meaning in terms of her experiences. I think it is understandable to want someone to take care of himself or herself by effectively telling them to clean up. But on the other hand it is also useful to think about what that person is perceiving, experiencing and communicating. It is also useful to be mindful of the fact that we are often more likely to remind women, rather than men, of the importance of looking after their appearance.

Moira appeared slow in her movements yet her anxiety could be clearly observed. At the prospect of picking up a cup, for example, Moira would stand, encircle her hands and breathe rapidly. My immediate reaction was to want to try to pick up the object she wanted so as to relieve her anxiety. I felt physically anxious and helpless watching her in this stuck position. I also felt angry and frustrated that she didn't get a move on.

In her notes, Moira was described as suffering from depression with psychotic features, and anxiety. Bodily aspects of her depression were clearly documented. She was described as prone to overeating and to neglecting herself by not washing. It was recorded that following the birth of her first child, at the age of eighteen in 1961, she was diagnosed as suffering from post-natal depression. Moira's notes detailed several more different diagnoses all relating to depression. At the age of forty, following a sterilisation, for example, Moira was told she was suffering from reactive depression. Subsequently, this changed to clinical depression. Her most recent diagnosis was bipolar II, whereby hypomania episodes have occurred with major recurrent depression, but mania has not.

When I interviewed Moira, I asked her about her background and about how she felt generally. Initially, she appeared very distracted. She told me she intended to go to the town hall after the interview to see who had died in her house. Moira described how she felt a presence of something like a spirit. 'It disturbs me, I'm sure it's somebody who used to live in my house and died there.' She asked me to describe again what my research was about. 'I hate my body', she stated in response. 'My body has deadness inside, the doctors tell me that's quite a common symptom in depression.' I then felt blank, as she seemed to stop dead in her tracks. I felt I couldn't say anything for a little while.

After staring at the floor, Moira announced that her mother suffered from paranoid schizophrenia and alcoholism. She proceeded to tell me that her childhood was very difficult. It seemed that her mother's problems developed when Moira was about five. She had a sister who was two years younger. Her mother was frequently taken into hospital and given, as Moira put it, 'weird treatments'. Moira said that she discovered several years later from her aunt, that her mother was treated with ECT. According to Moira, this treatment was sometimes effective, but her mother would always be readmitted to hospital within a short time. 'These were the days before drugs for schizophrenia', she said. Moira seemed to suggest that she was responsible for her mother's illness: 'It was all my fault, I think I was too much for anyone to cope with.'

While at home, Moira's mother's behaviour was very erratic. 'You couldn't tell whether she was coming or going.' At times, especially after a drink, she would become aggressive. Moira stated: 'She used to beat us up with a shovel, belt and poker, never her hands.' She went on to describe how she could never touch her mother as she was 'far away and frightening'. Moira also stated that her mother never touched her. I was struck by Moira's descriptions of the objects her mother used to beat her and her sister. Her statement 'never her hands', seemed an attempt to separate the objects used and her mother. It felt that Moira couldn't bear to think that her mother actually beat her, it was, rather, the objects. On the other hand, her mother's hands would have also meant that Moira received some physical contact.

Her father left when she was seven to live with another woman. Moira felt that as a result of this, her mother 'became more distressed than ever'. She was placed into foster care with her sister. As her aunt had six children of her own, she therefore couldn't help. However, she continued to visit Moira and her sister, and their foster family. Moira described how her foster family were 'pleasant enough' but she never felt really wanted. 'It wasn't like having a real mum and dad.' However, Moira started to feel closer to her foster mother at the time she left home. At eighteen, Moira got married. According to Moira, this was when her problems really began.

Her husband was ten years older: 'a real charmer, I couldn't believe my luck'. At first she thought he was pushy and rather outgoing. He always seemed to complain about other people doing wrong to him; he, of course was never to blame. He then started to accuse her of having lovers. 'He used to say the bed was warm.' 'Has someone been screwing you?', he would say. Then one evening after a night out with some of his friends, he hit her. Moira described how she felt shocked and tried to put it out of her mind. But the violence continued. Moira's apparent 'accidents' and bruises concerned her foster mother. Although her foster mother was a support, Moira couldn't tell her about the violence: 'I kept thinking it was my fault and that if I was nice he'd stop.' Moira's husband then stopped her seeing her foster mother. She stated that in those days there were no hostels for battered women: 'There was no help then, I suffered in silence.'

Moira stated that she rarely discussed having children with her husband. In fact, she thought they were never going to have any. She said she never really wanted children but ended up pregnant because her husband forced himself upon her at 'risky times of the month'. He refused to wear condoms. Moira decided to use the so-called 'safe' or 'rhythm method', 'but he forced himself on me at a risky time of the month and I fell pregnant'. She thought of using the cap, but decided against it because it meant she had to ask her husband if they were going to make love or not.

Her first daughter was particularly difficult to look after. Moira stated she couldn't cope with her as she cried constantly. Her husband would say, 'Do something with her'. Moira's daughter would only stop crying while being cuddled by her mother. But Moira said she couldn't cuddle her all the time. 'I didn't have magic powers.' She described how she felt very isolated at this time. All her friends suggested that she was 'independent' as she was also working as a secretary in a solicitor's office at the time. However, Moira found this hard work very tiring. Her second daughter was born a year later. 'She was no trouble at all. She was quiet and still, I had to check her to see if she was breathing.'

Moira's marriage eventually broke up when her husband met another woman. She described how he got custody of the children when he remarried. At the time, she attempted to reveal her husband's violence towards her. However, according to Moira, nobody believed her. 'They saw me as this nutter who couldn't command her life. He told the authorities that I was a neglectful mother and they believed him.' Her husband's new wife apparently couldn't cope with Moira's children. Moira said that both daughters were disturbed and both ended up in care. I asked her if she sees her daughters now. She replied that she occasionally sees the older one who now suffers from bi-polar psychosis. The second daughter doesn't want to know: 'There are two nutters in the family', she apparently says of her mother and sister.

Moira described to me her first overdose. 'It wasn't an overdose', she asserted. Her husband presented it that way. It occurred when her eldest daughter had just been born. According to Moira, she just took two sleeping pills, 'strong ones'. She said she was desperate for sleep. A sleep period of more than a mere two or three hours would sort her out, she thought. Her daughter wouldn't settle and she was at her wits end. Her husband took her to hospital because, as he told the hospital, he couldn't wake Moira up. 'Everyone thought I'd taken an overdose.' The doctors gave her a stomach pump and asked her lots of questions. Moira described how she felt that they were telling her off for 'causing all this fuss'. They appeared angry with her, she said. Moira spoke of these events in an anxious, trembling voice and told me about her frustration at this time: 'They said I was depressed. I couldn't convince them. I couldn't tell anyone my husband hit me. I needed help with my daughter, she wouldn't stop crying.' In response to Moira's account of events I began to feel physically anxious. I felt that she was trying desperately to convince me.

Moira described another incident when she had been at home with her first daughter. She had finally settled her and took a walk around the block by herself to settle herself. 'My husband came home and informed the social services.' Moira stated how she felt betrayed by him. He'd been in the Army and was very strict. 'Where have you been?', he said. Her husband did not support her, Moira said, when she was exhausted. 'Caring for the children was all my responsibility. My tiredness didn't matter to him. He just said I was a bad mother because I wasn't perfect and I didn't have magic powers.'

Moira said she didn't feel hopeful for the future. She had a boyfriend who she has been with for twenty-seven years. Although, according to Moira, he hasn't really been there for her. He is currently living in Jamaica, she told me. 'I haven't seen him since May, he's got another woman.'

A familiar experience for Moira it seemed, both her father and husband found other women, which left her distressed. 'My boyfriend says he wants friendship only', Moira stated. She described how she felt bitter and hurt. He apparently makes numerous excuses why Moira cannot go to Jamaica. 'I can't take it', she stated, 'this situation leads to me taking an overdose. My doctor thinks it would be a mistake to go to Jamaica'. Moira told me her doctor says it is time to move on: 'I can't move on – move on to what?' She spoke of going to Jamaica and how this might be a useful way to resolve things. 'Maybe I should go to Jamaica and confront him.' Moira said she would regret it if it didn't work out with her boyfriend. She would ask him, she said, if she goes, to keep the other woman out of the way. 'I might go for her – this has happened so many times.' Moira proceeded to tell me about other previous relationships where the men have had other women as well as her. 'I'm stuck on my boyfriend in Jamaica.' In response, I felt stuck too, and irritated. I felt the need to ask Moira to talk about something else. Somehow, I wanted to resolve this for her. I experienced a weary image of a record going round and round. It was similar to the frustration I felt when Moira's physical movements appeared to be stuck when she was about to do something such as pick up a cup. I felt the same need to get things going.

I proceeded to ask Moira how she felt about looking in the mirror. 'I feel angry and ugly', she stated, 'I hardly look in the mirror except when I'm doing my hair and make-up, and that's rare'. She described how she has a mirror in the bathroom but hates it. 'If I take a glimpse I feel ugly and old. People say I look younger than I am, but I feel old.' Moira went on to describe how she felt 'fat and frumpy'. 'People think I eat too much and that I eat all day, but I don't.' At this point, I felt compelled to ask Moira how she felt on the *inside*, but she continued to describe how she felt others saw her. She continued to describe how she felt ugly and how she felt other people thought she was greedy. 'I dress badly, and I look terrible', she stated. Again I was looking for the inside. However, what I experienced was perhaps this person presenting me with the inside out.

Moira stated that advertisements and magazines containing pictures of women made her feel worse. 'They make me feel overweight and as if I eat all day long, and that everything is my fault', she stated. 'I'm not happy with my big boobs. I'd like a flat stomach. My legs are better as they are toned, a result of me going to the gym. I always hated my big boobs. Even when I was slim, men commented on my big breasts, it was uncomfortable.' I asked Moira if there was a time in her life when she felt better about herself. 'At sixteen I was slim', she replied, 'I lost weight, I was seven stone. After I was sterilised at forty I started to put on weight'. She stated that she got herself sterilised so she would 'never worry about getting pregnant again'. She also appeared to go off sex at this time. For the past eighteen years, she said, she has put on weight, and has felt less like sex.

I asked Moira how she would like to be seen by the world. 'I'd like people to know I'm not a slob. There was a man on a bus who said, "get your fat bum out of my face". I eat an average amount of food.' With Moira's statements I began to feel increasingly deadened and cut off. I felt she was serving me up something cold with no life in it. I felt she was trying to articulate her needs but had got stuck. Her self-derogatory statements made me irritated. 'What can I do about it?', I thought. I felt that everything was stuck inside her. As I stated, I had attempted to ask Moira how she felt inside but she continued to describe what she looked like physically. I was interested in asking how she felt inside and how her distress might be communicated through her body. However, I got the strong feeling that her body *was her distress.*

When Moira talked about her body, she adopted popular discourses of femininity. It was as if she only had this language – these popular discourses – to describe how she felt about herself. She appeared to measure herself against popular images of female bodily perfection and view herself critically as if from outside. I thought that perhaps she could only give signs of how she felt in her gestures and not directly in language. Therefore, the observation of these gestures is important for staff who work with distressed women. On reflection, I considered Freud's important contention about the body as a language. In this context, the body is a series of signs relating to the individual's conflicts and experiences. The feminist theorists, Kristeva and Irigaray, also state how women suffer in their bodies. According to these theorists, women are not positioned within the realm of the symbolic, or rather the realm of speech and subjectivity. There has, indeed, been a large amount of literature focusing upon women's speech and the issue of women not being heard. As Deborah Cameron states, women are neither seen nor heard and their speech is often defined in a belittling way, as gossip, bitching, nagging, chitchat and so on (1985: 91). If women are not heard, how do they speak their suffering? Is it unspoken and unnameable? If this is the case, then it is only through gesture that the woman can communicate her distress. In light of these ideas, awareness of women's bodily presentation is important.

It is also vital to pay attention to bodily responses, as they perhaps indicate the experiences of the people we work with. My feelings of deadness, of being stuck and of frustration, perhaps indicate Moira's experiences in her life. She had received little physical contact when young and perhaps she had deadened herself to avoid feeling the need for this. Her weight, her feelings of being dead inside and her self-neglect by not washing might have indicated this. These actions might also have been attempts at putting other people off. It seemed from Moira's account of the people she had loved, that she had been let down by them. Perhaps she had subsequently made a point – perhaps unconsciously – to prevent being attractive to, and wanted by, other people. 'There's no point looking nice', she said at the end of our time together. It was somehow gratifying for her to put people off. But what was very clear to me, and this is something I felt very moved by, was her need of people that she vehemently denied through her defensive presentation.

I also felt struck by the hard physical work Moira had done as a wife and a mother. She had never felt good enough in these roles. She had also experienced domestic violence, which clearly contributed to her feelings of depression. The writing of the second wave feminists, which I have detailed in Chapter 4, state how women's roles and, consequently, their hard physical work as wives and mothers, often lead them to become mentally distressed. These theories, often seen as not relevant to the lives of women today living in the supposed post-feminist ages, clearly are still important. In my interactions with Moira, I felt these theories could be directly applied to her situation.

## Alice

Alice, who was forty-eight, attended the day hospital twice a week for support for her drinking and depression. She looked at me intensely when she approached me about my research: 'I don't like looking in the mirror', she said, 'it hurts me'. Despite this she said she thought it would be 'helpful to talk', as that was what she did every week with her psychiatrist. Another reason for seeing her psychiatrist was because she had taken an overdose very recently. Alice told me she had been depressed for two years and had taken thirteen overdoses during that period. Her family had always notified the hospital, she said. Her weekly sessions with the psychiatrist also meant that she was only given her medication, which she took daily, on a weekly basis. She told me that she also heard voices. This was detailed in her notes as most likely to occur as a result of acute stress.

In her notes it was also recorded that Alice was diagnosed with depression, alcohol abuse and possibly a personality disorder. She was described as having no motivation at all when depressed. She was also described as neglecting her self-care at these times. She would not wash, she said, and couldn't be bothered to go to the hairdresser. Her husband frequently took over the cleaning and other household tasks when Alice was ill. However, he was rather reluctant to do this. According to Alice, he would be irritated with her and remind her frequently that domestic tasks were *her* role, not his. One of the symptoms that had been recorded in her notes, as indicative of her depression, was 'a lack of interest in household tasks'.

I was rather hesitant about interviewing Alice because of her recent attempt to end her life. I spoke to her psychiatrist, expressing my concern. Her psychiatrist suggested that I shouldn't be too concerned by her presentation. They stated that she had a personality disorder meaning that her problem was behavioural rather than due to a specific mental illness.

I asked them to say more about this. One of the features of personality disorder, they pointed out, is the manipulation of other people. Consequently, they said, she was keen to latch on to as many people as possible to get their attention.

Alice was extremely polite to me and seemed to want to go out of her way to fit in with my availability for the interview. We agreed a time and she thanked me, stating she was very grateful for my time and interest in her. She asked me again what my research was about. In response she exclaimed that she hated her face and her body, but it would help to talk about it with somebody. She stated that her psychiatrist always seems to know how she feels without her saying anything. 'He knows I wear a mask', she stated putting her hand over her face. 'I'm smiling', she said, 'but he seems to know that I'm depressed underneath'. Did anyone else know this, I asked. She replied that nobody else seemed to know; she wears the mask well.

In terms of her bodily presentation and appearance, Alice was of average height and quite bulky and heavy. She seemed to walk in a stiff, controlled way. Alice did not seem to mix with the other women at the day hospital, who, as I stated earlier, formed a group in the seating area. Alice, instead, tended to walk around or sit by herself. I observed that when she sat down she proceeded to rub the top of her legs as if trying to soothe herself. This had a soothing effect on me and I wondered if she was trying to calm those around her. When I interviewed Alice, my thoughts about her trying to soothe others seemed to make sense. She told me about her violent feelings about herself and subsequent attacks upon her body.

Alice said that she was born in Africa and came to this country with her parents in the 1950s. She described herself as 'British Black'. Alice's mother, while pregnant with her, experienced some pregnancy complications. 'She was never very well when I was young.' Alice stated that she felt she had done something wrong but couldn't work out what. 'My mother seemed cross with me. I was the youngest. I thought you were spoiled being the youngest.' Following Alice's birth the family moved to England. Alice was never told why this decision was made. She guessed it was something to do with her father's work. 'Maybe he didn't work before I don't remember, but he became a cleaner in a local school.' Alice said that in the 1950s, when her family moved, there were not many black people in this country. 'Not like there are now', she said. Alice described how she remembered how her mother appeared to feel ashamed of the family. 'I always thought she was embarrassed by us – me, my brother and my sister.'

Alice said she felt very isolated as a child. She found it difficult to make friends. All the other girls, she told me, seemed to form groups and all got on well together. She was the only black child in her class, she said, and was consequently called names. 'When I got to primary school', she stated, 'I was called blackie, golliwog'. I found, in response to these comments, that I felt attacked and violated by Alice and this made me feel uneasy. I wondered whether Alice was unconsciously trying to make me feel I was one of her attackers. Consequently, this made me feel uncomfortable, so I then felt I was being attacked.

Alice said that she was taken into care intermittently during the first ten years of her life. I asked why this happened and she replied, 'My mum had complications with her pregnancy'. I was struck by the detached way in which Alice said this. It was as if her mother's pregnancy had nothing to do with her presence in the world. She added that she kept in touch with her mother who had died a year ago. Her mother, according to Alice, was very old fashioned and strict. She stated again that she couldn't work out what she had done wrong. 'Mum was angry with me and I couldn't ask why.' Alice stated that she was unable to tell her mother anything. 'I did some terrible things', she said. 'I feel things have been my fault.' Alice began to rub the top of her legs and rocked backwards and forwards. As mentioned above, I found this action rather soothing and almost hypnotising. I started to feel rather sleepy and cut off. I realised that this action was perhaps Alice's attempt to soothe us both in preparation for what she was about to say.

'I don't deserve to be happy', she said. 'I want to die before I'm fifty and I think I'm a bitch.' I felt rather attacked by these statements and began to feel dizzy. 'You see, I've done some terrible things.' Alice described how she had been raped at the age of seventeen. She was still living with her parents at this time. Things were very strained at home, she said. 'I couldn't talk to my mum and dad, so I spent a lot of time in my room.' There was one of her dad's friends in the house a lot. 'He always seemed drunk to me', Alice said. She found this man attractive and used to flirt with him. 'That got me out of my room', she stated. Then he started to come to their house while her parents were out. One night, Alice said he came round and 'started being over friendly'. Alice said, 'I let myself get raped by him'. I had the sensation that she wanted me to feel the way she did. I experienced the need to tell her that, of course, she was not to blame, but I ended by feeling helpless. I found her presence rather overwhelming and felt rather crowded out. I found myself asking – and I felt rather detached from myself – if she was able to tell her mother about this incident. 'Of course not!', I found myself thinking before she made a reply. I felt she was in an impossible situation. My responses were quite correct. Alice said she couldn't tell her parents because they would have handled it so badly, they certainly wouldn't have given her any support, she said. 'They couldn't manage, my mum couldn't have managed me, it's too heavy', she said, as if referring to herself.

Alice then proceeded to tell me that four years later she was raped again. This time it was by a stranger in a street. 'I let it happen again', she stated.

Alice found that she was pregnant and had an abortion. She couldn't afford to go private, she said. The doctor was not sympathetic. 'She implied that it was all my fault, and, yes, it was, but I did need some help then.' Alice didn't tell anyone about the abortion, except her sister. After these two events, Alice said she 'fell into a depression'. She couldn't stop crying, she said, and found it difficult to look after herself. She said she just ate rubbish and didn't drink properly. At this time, she felt that her insides were rotting. She had apparently asked her GP for an x-ray to prove she was right. The GP laughed at her, she said. 'How would you be alive if your insides were rotting?', he had asked.

In addition, Alice stated that she either stopped washing herself altogether or washed herself too much. She explained that she now understood this excessive washing as an attempt to cleanse herself after the rapes. However, she said she did not understand this at the time and became aware of it only after watching a TV programme about the subject. At the time, her doctor told her to look after herself better. 'I couldn't quite get it right. I either didn't care or went over the top.' She was prescribed antidepressants but was not offered any other support. Alice stated that she still hadn't told anyone about the rapes. She suggested that her doctor should have known about her distress perhaps, I thought when she said this, by looking behind her mask.

At the age of twenty-two, Alice met her husband. She was working at a library at this time. 'I quite enjoyed it, the peace and quiet, I was not bothered by anyone.' Her husband was a fellow worker and as Alice described him, rather quiet and calm himself. Her husband seemed to be happy to support her, she said. She didn't tell him much about her background, including the rapes. Over the years they had five children. I wondered how Alice felt about sex in relation to these experiences, but I felt it was not quite right to ask Alice about this issue, as it may be too personal.

There was a son of twenty-six, twin girls who were twenty-four, and two more boys aged sixteen and eleven. Alice stated that she took on the main responsibility of caring for her children while her husband supported her financially. 'I was bought up to believe that a woman should always please her husband, to do the housework and do everything properly.' Alice stated that she believed that she failed at this. 'I'm not a good mother and I'd be better out of the way.' She said that her children are all grown up and live at home. They all contribute to the cooking and housework. 'They all like it, but I'm not sure that they should do it, I should do it.' One of her daughters is a paranoid schizophrenic and is frequently in hospital when she doesn't take her medication. Alice said she feels guilty about this, 'I'm not well enough to look after her, and I feel I'm just a burden to her, to all of them'. At this point Alice's mobile phone rang. 'I'm talking at the moment, I'll call you back, I'm alright', she said to him. 'That's my husband', she told me, 'he's always checking up on me'. It seemed that

Alice's depression was a cause for concern for her family. She described how when she 'gets suicidal' they hide her tablets so she cannot find them.

I asked Alice how she felt about looking in the mirror. She had mentioned her feelings about looking in the mirror before I interviewed her. This time she went into more detail. She described how she often covers up the mirror in her bedroom (her husband, she said, insisted upon having a full length one in the bedroom) because it speaks to her. Alice explained that she hears voices and she hears them when she looks at her reflection in the mirror. She stated that she hears a well-spoken man or woman who are her teachers from school. According to Alice, these voices say she is 'evil and a black bitch'. She said, 'I look in the mirror and it says I'm a black bastard. I look ugly and fat'. Alice also described how as she walks along the street people whisper to her. 'They say the same things as the mirror – that I'm fat, ugly and evil.' She then described how when she looks in the mirror, she hears the names she was called while at school. 'The mirror calls me those names too – the same names I was called at school because I was the only black kid.'

Alice stated that two years ago she had her first admission to a psychiatric ward. She had taken an overdose and was hearing these distressing voices. She was given a medication called Clozaril. This particular medication requires that the patient have regular blood tests to carefully monitor the medication levels. When she was discharged, she took an overdose of Clozaril and she was told this attempt was almost fatal. Following this occasion, she has taken ten more overdoses, but her husband always finds her in time, she said. She is now prescribed an anti-depressant medication, an anti-psychotic medication, and a medication to help her sleep. Alice stated that she had been told that medication would eventually cause harm to her internal organs. 'I'm glad about this', she said, 'it means there is harm being done to me'. I felt a sense of hopelessness in response to these statements. It also made me angry with her and I was beginning to feel worn out.

I asked Alice to describe how her body made her feel – happy or unhappy? Alice told me that she drinks alcohol and cuts her arms to feel better. 'I don't deserve to feel better', she stated. She said she wanted to be out of the way. 'I sometimes look as if I'm happy and smiling, but underneath I'm very depressed.' She went on to say how cutting her arms feels satisfactory because it's a way of punishing herself, 'for all the bad things I have done'. Alice also described how she drinks too much alcohol. 'The penalty for drinking too much is to get fat', she said. At this point Alice seemed to state this penalty was inevitable. She stated how she has a hangover almost every day. 'I feel disgusted with myself', she said, 'I am a drunk'. Alice explained that she was drinking heavily while in hospital during her last admission. 'It got me into trouble', she said. Alice explained that she becomes sexually active when she is drunk. She stated that she had no wish to stop drinking because it made her relaxed. 'I'm excessive and end up in bed with someone.' She then stated that she is vulnerable at these times but also in control. 'When I am drunk, I can cope with anything, I feel I can cope with anything because I am not thinking.'

I asked how Alice expressed her feelings and she replied that she thought she did while drunk because she doesn't check herself at those times. She said that 'there is room for improvement, I put myself down, but I'm really not a good wife. I should do more things around the house and not leave it to my husband and children'. She explained that she finds it difficult to express her feelings. Her feelings didn't really matter, she said, she had let everyone down. Alice stated how she always tried to be good, but had allowed herself to do terrible things. She went on to talk about washing herself. When she doesn't go to church she washes herself more than necessary. Then Alice announced that she sometimes rubs herself with bleach. Although I had heard this from previous patients I had worked with, I nevertheless felt shocked. 'I really want to be clean', Alice said. 'The mirror calls me a black bastard.' At this point I asked Alice how she wanted to be seen by the outside world. She replied that she wanted to look less scruffy and said she wanted to dress better. 'I have difficulty getting up in the morning, I always look dirty and scruffy', she stated. 'I would like to be seen as a caring mother and wife. I'm not really into fashion. But I would like to look nice for the family. I'd like to be someone who can be trusted and approached easily.'

During our conversations, Alice stated that she was 'not there', or 'invisible'. 'I'm a wife', she said, 'but I'm not really there, nobody sees me'. I wondered if this related to her feelings of being a black woman, and in addition to this, a black female patient. Alice pointed out frequently during our interactions that I was in physical opposition to her, being tall. This made me wonder whether she was implying that I had stature and therefore status, and was consequently visible. I considered that her comments also implied that as a person with a mental illness she was invisible, whereas as a 'sane' *and white* person I was visible.

During my contact with Alice, the word 'guilt' came to my mind frequently. I felt that she was telling me how guilty she felt. It was as if she had felt guilty from the time of her birth. Her mother had had pregnancy complications while carrying her. Alice seemed to believe that these were somehow her fault and it meant that her mother couldn't look after her – hence her subsequent foster care. Because of her feelings of guilt, it seemed that Alice wished to attack her body as a punishment. This was apparent in her wish to kill herself and her self-harm.

I felt that Alice projected her guilt onto others, which returned in the form of hearing voices from outside. Alice also attacked her black skin by excessively washing and sometimes cleaning herself with bleach. It seemed that she had internalised the guilt she had understood her mother to be feeling when the family first moved to this country. I felt she attacked and violated me in her comments. I wondered if this was my defence against not wanting to feel like her attacker. Consequently, in defence, I felt that I was the one being attacked. Alice also attacked herself for what she perceived as failing as a wife and mother. The pressure to perform well in these roles was particularly strong in her upbringing. She felt violent against herself for failing and this revealed itself in her bodily expressions of self-harm.

## The gendered body

There is a wealth of writings on the body in terms of gendered identity. This book has focused on the body particularly in relation to the experience of psychosis. I devoted a chapter to women's experience of mental illness (and the ways in which psychiatry has sought to control the female body). I have not provided much information on men's embodied experience of mental illness (except in the two case studies presented above). Nor have I given attention to the experiences of various 'sexualities' (e.g. transsexualism, transgenderism, bisexuality and so on), which, of course, relate to the experience of 'being in a body'. It is less than thirty years since these 'forms' of sexuality were presented in the American DSM (Diagnostic and Statistical Manual of Mental Disorder) as psychiatric conditions. Homosexuality was removed from the DSM in the 1970s. It seems that remnants of the view that homosexuality constitutes a mental disorder still remain in mental health practice today.[1]

I have suggested that mental health practitioners are often inclined to consider the mentally ill body in biomedical terms. I have stated that Foucault's insights are useful here. The body is a rather passive entity in Foucault's estimation. It is controlled, trained, moulded and so on, to fit in with and reflect prevailing ideas. Dominant forms of knowledge about mental illness bear upon the bodies of those who receive a psychiatric diagnosis, rendering them to be considered as biological subjects. In his discussion of psychiatric discourse and bodies, Foucault is not gender specific and, as we have seen, he has been accused of being rather gender blind. However, his concept of discourse and the body is useful in understanding the differing experiences of the sexes.

In my observations of, and interviews with, patients there were clear differences between the men and women. The men were much more willing to come forward. It did occur to me that perhaps the men thought my research might be rather saucy considering it was about the body. Leaving this point aside, it did seem to me that the men felt important enough to be considered. It seemed that they were not at all phased by something as concrete as the body. They appeared to speak relatively freely about their, albeit distressing, bodily experiences. However, it is worth noting that just because the men seemed to find the words to talk about their experiences, this does not mean that they found it an easy process.

The women were much more reluctant to participate. I was eager to ask them how they felt on the *inside* and to consider how their distress was reflected or communicated on the *outside*. The women seemed to focus upon the outside, particularly in terms of their attractiveness. Cultural pressures and discourses of ideal physical perfection seemed to influence and affect them more strongly than the men. It seemed that when these women talked about their bodies they adopted popular discourses of femininity, as I have said, as if this was the only way of talking about themselves. As a result of such expectations, women are particularly watchful of their bodies and looking pretty and so on is necessary to their feelings of well-being. I found their self-deprecating comments rather deadening and irritating. I considered, however, that these statements were possible metaphors for the way women feel about themselves in relation to the world. The use of metaphor, however, implies there is a 'real' or exact way of expressing something.

In Chapter 1, I asked the question of how is distress communicated through language. According to the theorists Kristeva and Irigaray, which I discussed in Chapter 6, women suffer in their bodies in their position outside the realm of speech. Is it therefore the case that women are required to adopt a language in order to communicate their distress? The language available to the women I observed and interviewed was one of self-deprecation, which was apparent in the way they compared themselves unfavourably with 'ideals' of female appearance and behaviour. It is also worth noting that all people, whether male or female, who enter the psychiatric system lose their sense of identity, and certainly as a speaking subject.

The women appeared worried that I wouldn't want to interview them as they felt they were too unattractive or didn't dress well and so forth. Was it that they thought I would compare their bodies to mine and somehow criticise them? I felt I needed to approach the women much more carefully and sensitively than the men. When they began to form a group within the day hospital, I felt they were more comfortable and appeared more able to express themselves more freely with each other. When I participated within this group they seemed more comfortable in asking me about my research and, subsequently, some of the women expressed an interest in taking part. Perhaps this indicates the need for allowing women to have some secure space within clinical practice, so that they may feel more able to express themselves.

Do mental health practitioners inevitably consider their women patients' bodies in terms of attractiveness? We can certainly say that within Western culture, women are reduced to bodies. Sandra Bartky, for example, condemns the sexual objectification of the female body. This brings about, as Bartky puts it, the 'degrading identity of a person with her body' (1990:

23). Of course, the very term 'objectification' conjures up images for most of us of oppression. It is important, however, to question how far the experience of objectification contributes to psychological oppression.

In mental health practice, I think it can be said that much emphasis is placed on women's bodies in terms of their mental wellness. It is often presumed that if a woman *looks* better she will *feel* better, and frequently this is, indeed, the case. But it is worth considering that when a woman is tiresomely preoccupied with her appearance she might be saying something about her experiences. For the women in my study, it seemed that their distress was stuck inside and that their bodies were their distress. I mentioned to a member of staff at the day hospital that the women's distress appeared stuck inside of them. She agreed and said, 'It's a matter of getting it out'. Perhaps it's a matter of acknowledging and respecting the distress even if it still remains inside and appears unspoken.

As I stated in Chapter 3, there has been an increase in the last decade in the numbers of young men killing themselves, and there has also been an increase in the prevalence of eating disorders in men. Entering the psychiatric system has consequences for male embodiment. For men, anti-psychotic medication, for example, brings about erectile and ejaculatory dysfunction, decreased sexual desire (which also affects women) and growth of breast tissue. It is also considered that schizophrenic men are less interested than 'non-schizophrenic' men in forming sexual relationships. This is thought to severely affect their self-esteem as culturally they are generally expected, to a large extent, to initiate sexual relationships. The effect of mental illness and psychiatric care on men and their bodies requires much attention. Whether working with men or women, we could consider the body as a kind of clinical 'tool' as well as a clinical object. We talk about patients' appearance, sexualise and objectify their bodies. On the other hand, we can make room to consider the body as a way in to understanding the experiences of the person who lives it.

## Conclusion

I have presented two women patients I observed and interviewed at a day hospital. I was surprised by their reluctance to come forward and their impression that, although I wanted to talk to women about their bodies, I was somehow only interested in women who felt great about themselves and their bodies. I felt that these women, perhaps, did not feel I wanted to consider them and hear what they had to say. It was certainly true that they were self-deprecating about themselves as women, particularly in their perceived failure as mothers and carers, and in terms of their physical appearance.

I considered that my bodily responses were also important for me to understand and make sense of. I felt that these were clues to what the women were experiencing, such as in the case of Moira in particular, and my feeling of being physically stuck in response to her experience of being stuck in her current situation. An awareness of how the women related to my body was also important, as in the case of Alice who seemed to stand me in contrast to her in order to emphasise how invisible she felt.

I observed that the women used non-verbal language apparent in their bodily presentation and various gestures, to communicate their experiences. Both Moira and Alice seemed to be reluctant to take care of themselves in terms of washing and so forth. Although I felt rather compelled to tell them to do better in this area of their lives, I nevertheless considered that they might be communicating how they felt *inside*. I also felt that their gestures were clues to their lived experiences. Moira, for example, encircled her hands when she tried to do something as a possible indication of how stuck she felt. Alice had expressed her cultural experiences through her bodily presentation in her attempt to excessively clean herself, as she had perhaps internalised the difficulties her mother had experienced upon arriving in the UK. She would rub her legs to soothe us both in an attempt, I thought, to protect us from the badness she felt inside of her. As I have stated, the psychoanalytically orientated feminist theorists Irigaray and Kristeva, suggest that women's suffering is bodily as they are positioned outside the patriarchal realm of speech. With this in mind, it is vital for mental health practitioners to consider the meaning inherent in women's bodily gestures in terms of their experiences.

I greatly enjoyed being with the patients I have discussed in this chapter. They gave generously of their time and I hope I have been respectful in my presentations of them. As I have stated, I have only offered suggestions of what these patients' bodily presentation might indicate in terms of their life experiences. It did seem as if their symptoms were not meaningless and did not merely relate to universal diagnostic categories of mental illness. It seems that these patients' various 'symptoms' of mental illness in the form of seemingly 'bizarre' hallucinations and delusions did clearly relate to their experiences as people.

Turan's radioactive metal plate in his leg and his infected open wound, were real to him. I could not see them. But these 'symptoms' and their expression did not mean that he was *just* schizophrenic. As it turned out they symbolised something about his emotional needs. I was able to understand him better through paying attention to the meanings apparent in his expressions, particularly in relation to his upbringing as an orthodox Muslim and in terms of his rather difficult relationship with his parents. I therefore went beyond seeing him as a kind of biological subject. By attempting to make sense of my physical and psychical responses, I was able to consider how Turan was communicating his experiences to me. The recognition of a mental health patient as a person with needs and experiences. Isn't this what 'working therapeutically' as a mental health nurse is all about?

# Chapter 9

# Developing practice

In this chapter, I will identify ways in which awareness of patients' expression of their lived experience through their bodies – and staff responses to this – may be incorporated into mental health practice, so as to improve the quality of patient treatment and care. However, I will first summarise the themes I have outlined in this book. My focus throughout has been to stress the importance of mental health staff paying attention to the bodily presentation and appearance of their patients in a way that goes beyond attention to diagnosis and treatment. Bodily presentations might well be an indication of the patients' life experiences. In addition, the psychical and physical responses of mental health practitioners and the acknowledgement and understanding of these in working with patients, is also important in enabling them to better understand their patients' experiences and needs.

Chapter 2 defined and explored the concept of 'lived experience' and the 'lived body'. I argued that mainstream mental health practice, with its biomedical understanding of the cause, presentation and treatment of mental illness, often fails to acknowledge the life experiences of patients that are frequently expressed through their (bodily) symptoms. I also briefly outlined the philosophical tradition of phenomenology, which focuses upon experience, consciousness and relation to others, and in this context, I explored phenomenological perspectives, including Merleau-Ponty's concept of the 'lived body'. I also identified Freud's place in this tradition.

Chapter 3 explored Foucault's discussion of power and discourse and their effects upon the body. Prevailing discourses produce knowledge that is used to regulate and discipline the body. Therefore, according to Foucault, the body is a passive entity upon which prevailing discourses are inscribed. Applied to mental health practice, I argued that prevailing and dominant discourses about mental illness could influence the way we see mental health patients and their bodies. Mental health practitioners, within mainstream mental health practice, tend to see the bodily presentations of mental illness as relating to a specific diagnostic category with a biological cause. The bodily aspects of mental illness apparent in the patients I observed and interviewed in Chapter 8 were clearly detailed in their notes. There was a suggestion that their bodily presentations – including lack of self-care, low energy levels, or sleeplessness – were due to their clinical condition – depression, say, or psychosis. There seemed to be no further acknowledgement or examination of what their bodily presentations signified in terms of their lived experience.

I then outlined how psychiatry has understood and defined mental illness in relation to the body. Prevailing discourses about mental illness have focused upon biological causes such as brain chemical imbalances. Treatments for mental illness have consisted of biochemical and physical procedures such as ECT and psychotropic medication. Mental health professionals are also encouraged in their assessment of patients, to observe bodily signs, such as unusual clothing or gestures, which are considered as an indication of a specific mental illness. Mainstream mental health practice, therefore, tends to see the body and its presentation within a biomedical framework. This was also apparent in the patients described in Chapter 8. As I stated above, the bodily aspects of their mental illness were documented in their notes. Discussions of the bodily aspects of mental distress did not go beyond suggesting that these symptoms were the meaningless, biologically determined effect of their medically understood condition.

Chapter 4 explored feminist approaches to the body. I discussed how theories within second wave feminism have been applied to an understanding of women's mental distress. Socialist and Marxist feminism has understood women's oppression as stemming from their relationship to the economy and their roles within the family. Theorists, including Ann Oakley and Agnes Miles, state how these factors often contribute to women's mental distress. These ideas, although expressed in the 1970s, still ring true in broad terms today. The women I interviewed seemed to experience mental distress partly or wholly as a result of their roles as wives, carers and mothers. They considered themselves inadequate, appearing to be well aware of the prevailing discourses surrounding women's supposed 'natural' adoption of these roles. Their partners were often violent towards them and they often took on sole responsibility for the care of children and sick relatives. The body is relevant in this context because of the apparent impact of the hard physical work these women undertook in these roles, and how this affected their sense of self and their mental health.

I also outlined ideas regarding women's oppression within radical feminism. Radical feminist theorists have identified patriarchal structures that serve to control women's bodies and sexuality, and justify the position of women in certain 'female' roles. Writers such as Phyllis Chesler and Elaine Showalter have applied such ideas to the position of women within the psychiatric system. Physical interventions such as ECT, medication and leucotomies, according to these theorists, are mostly given to women in order to control their perceived wayward behaviour and sexuality.

Chapter 5 outlined Freud's writings on the body beginning with his theory of hysteria. It was my intention to outline Freud's extensive attention to the body and to apply aspects of these theories to the patients I observed and interviewed. Freud stated that the symptoms manifested in the body are significant in terms of the lived experience of individuals. He detailed the conflicts of his early women patients in terms of their domestic situation and their desire. These ideas are important because they imply that symptoms have specific meaning for each individual rather than relating to a diagnostic category. In the case of the women I interviewed, I felt that their bodily gestures communicated aspects of the conflicts in their lives. Moira's stuck position and the encircling of her hands, for example, seemed to reflect the way she seemed stuck in her life.

Freud also specifies the importance of the body in early development. The infant learns its separateness and identity through its relation to erotogenic zones on its body. Freud describes the sense of self, or ego, as developing from bodily sensations on the surface of the body and from identifications with those outside, particularly the primary carer. The patients I interviewed each seemed to have a sense of self that was fragile and fragmented, and this was often symbolised within their bodies. Tom's smashed up leg for example, which he clutched so tenderly, appeared to symbolise the smashed up and fragmented aspects of himself that he was attempting to hold together. In my countertransference responses to Tom and several other patients, I had a bodily sense of this when I felt dizzy and thrown off course. I wondered if this indicated these patients' lack of integration and cohesiveness.

In his admittedly sexist discussion of women's bodies in terms of penis envy, Freud has been largely criticised by feminist writers, as I outlined in Chapter 5, as being biologically determinist. However, in his early work with patients with hysteria, he clearly goes beyond biological explanations in his understanding of women's distress. He presents these early female patients in terms of their subjectivity and identifies the conflicts between their desire and their ties to domesticity. Therefore, Freud pays attention to the social situations of these women and the ways in which their conflicts were often manifested in their bodies.

Chapter 6 outlined theories about the body in psychosis. I began with the work of Schilder who suggests that a sense of body image is influenced by the amount of libidinal energy individuals invest in their bodies, and is reinforced and confirmed by their primary carer. Schilder suggests that in psychosis, individuals experience a lack of libidinal investment in their body and therefore a lack of interest in their body. This was apparent in the case of Tom, who appeared to feel detached from his body, or did not have a sense of his body, and clearly said he felt there was no life in it. In this context, it is unrealistic to expect patients to feel good about their bodies and to attend to their self-care. Perhaps staff would benefit from an awareness of a patient's experience of being detached from, or not owning their body. Furthermore, Schilder's insight goes beyond the suggestion within mental health practice that lack of self-care is a 'negative' symptom of schizophrenia along with a deadened affect, apathy and so forth.

Schilder also suggests that there is excessive introjection and projection in psychosis. Outside objects, for example, are often felt as part of the body image. I went on to outline the work of Lacan who specifies that in psychosis, the name-of-the-father is foreclosed, and subsequently stands in opposition to the individual. The individual, therefore, is still positioned in the pre-verbal, imaginary realm of trying to be the phallus in order to satisfy the mother's lack of it. In this context, the individual has not internalised and identified with the phallus or the name-of-the-father, and become a speaking 'I'. I felt with many of the patients that they did not experience a firm sense of identity, and that their speech was often deadened and lifeless.

The theorists Kristeva and Irigaray, suggest that women suffer within their bodies as they have limited access to patriarchal language, or rather the symbolic, in Lacanian terms. I had a sense of this when interacting with the women patients I observed in Chapter 8 and I felt their distress was rather stuck inside and they appeared to have limited means by which to express it. When the women spoke about their bodies, they adopted popular discourses of femininity and compared themselves negatively against them. Therefore, it seems that attention to bodily gestures in the case of women seems particularly important in the understanding of their distress.

The theories of Klein involve an understanding of the processes of splitting, projection and introjection in psychosis. For Klein, psychosis occurs when the individual remains or regresses to the paranoid–schizoid position where these processes are active. The ego is fragmented because of excessive splitting and parts of the self are projected out onto the figures of outside things or people. Several of the patients I interviewed appeared to project out parts of themselves, which returned in the form, for example, of persecutory voices from outside.

Chapter 7 first outlined Freud's theories on psychosis and the psychotic person's supposed reduced capacity for transference. Subsequent theorists following Klein have considered that psychotic people do, indeed, transfer or, rather, project their emotions onto the analyst. Theorists such as Winnicott and Searles acknowledge the difficulties involved in working with psychotic and borderline psychotic individuals, which I described in some of the interviews. I felt intruded upon, for example, by Turan's words, which I also felt got into me. Other theorists have discussed the importance of examining psychical and physical countertransference responses to patients in understanding of their experiences.

My observations of, and interviews with, the mental health patients detailed in Chapter 8, reveal ways in which a patient's lived experience may be expressed by bodily means. The body in this context is not merely an array of meaningless symptoms relating to a specific mental illness with a biological cause. To incorporate an emphasis upon the body in this context into mental health practice would require staff to focus upon the lived experiences of patients and the ways in which past and present experiences are often manifested in the body.

Gathering background details of patients is already an essential part of the assessment process carried out by staff when people with mental illness are initially admitted to in-patient mental health settings. As I have stated, attention is given to the bodily aspects of distress. However, I consider that increased attention to what patients' bodies signify in terms of their lived experience is necessary to understand them better. The question arises as to what staff might do with this increased awareness. In addition, there is the question of how awareness of the body and countertransference issues can be effectively incorporated into mental health practice. I will now offer some suggestions.

## Mental health nursing practice

In this book, I have attempted to convey how a range of theoretical perspectives can help inform the practitioner's understanding about the ways in which a person with psychosis might experience the world around them. For nurses to be aware of the importance of paying attention to patients' bodily presentation and the countertransference responses these evoke, an awareness of the theories supporting these phenomena needs to be incorporated into mental health nurse training. Nurses are currently taught Freud's main theories in terms of his concept of dreams, the unconscious and so forth. However, his extensive attention to the body as language and in terms of its importance in early development is not examined. As I have stated, there is currently much attention to the body within mental health practice, particularly in relation to the assessment process. The perspectives outlined in this book might usefully add to these understandings. They may enable the mental health practitioner, supported by a theoretical base, to go beyond diagnosis and attend more closely to the experiences of the people they care for. This approach would add to the current commitment to, and emphasis upon, patient-centred care within mental health nursing practice.

If we are to think about what a person might be communicating through their bodily symptoms, in particular, it is necessary to consider their needs and experiences and this requires time and energy. It might be the case that nurses would be reluctant to think about the body as a vital communicator of life experience. They may state that there is not enough time for this process. Mental health nurses, in my experience, frequently express frustration about reduced numbers of staff, too much paperwork and so on. It can also be rather overwhelming to think about the needs of people we care for, as their experiences are often painful and traumatic. Perhaps it is easier to consider psychiatric symptoms within a biomedical framework. Stating that a person's distress is all due to brain chemicals requires less attention to details. Yet, in doing this, we are not considering the patients we work with as people with needs and experiences; we are merely reducing them to biological 'subjects'.

The mental health nurse's role is multiple and unique. I think that nurses are in a privileged position that other professionals do not share to the same extent. In their daily practice, nurses perform seemingly mundane tasks. They sit with patients often for long periods, particularly when carrying out close observations. Nurses wait with patients when they attend appointments. On a ward setting, nurses are there when patients eat their meals and are there during the night. They open the curtains in the morning. They make conversation with patients and often spend time with them in silence. In a more senior capacity, nurses supervise other staff to carry out these tasks.

In terms of their unique role, mental health nurses are often perceived as adhering to a biomedical approach to patient care (Hamblet 2000). Nurses are, indeed, uniquely responsible for the administration (and psychiatrists, at least at present, for the prescribing) of medication, including anti-psychotics, mood stabilisers and anti-depressants. The nurse's role will also overlap with other mental health practitioners such as social workers and occupational therapists. In the context of both a ward setting and a community mental health team, for example, nurses will address social issues including housing, family interventions, relapse prevention and so forth. However, as a challenge to the biomedical framework, there is another role that is particular to mental health nursing that is often overlooked within mental health services, which is initiating a therapeutic relationship with patients.

## Working therapeutically

The idea of 'working therapeutically', although fundamental to mental health nursing practice, is often difficult to define. However, it can be stated that mental health nurses have the unique role – which is also a central component of the therapeutic relationship – of *being with* patients. In this context, the nurse's role is to create a secure base whereby the patient can explore and communicate their feelings and experiences. The nurse will, therefore, be with the patient in a respectful, considerate and trustworthy way and consequently, 'contain' the patient's distress, which means enabling the patient to feel secure and safe. This process involves the nurse staying with the patient in their distress by experiencing and reflecting upon it. Consequently, as Watkins points out, the patient 'learns that intense feelings, fears and fantasies can be contained, reflected upon and made sense of' (Watkins 2001: 156). The nurse–patient relationship is therefore understood as a relationship, and is about 'being' rather than 'doing'. In their privileged role, the mental health nurse is in an ideal position to think about and explore the meanings inherent in the often-bodily symptoms of patients that go beyond attention to diagnosis. However, nurses are often very caught up with 'doing'. There is a clear emphasis within mental health nursing practice upon action plans and outcomes, and risk and its prevention. These factors tend to reduce the quality time nurses spend with patients and focus very much on *doing.*

In this book, I have suggested that as mental health practitioners we could look beyond diagnosis and think about what our patients are experiencing and how their seemingly meaningless symptoms often relate to their life events and often symbolise the ways in which, as individuals, they are relating to and experiencing the world. This, of course, requires thinking. Nurses, of course, do think, but are not encouraged to do so. It is often frightening to think about our patients and even more frightening to take note of the impact they often have upon us. We are frequently overwhelmed by our patients' often fragmented and disturbing experiences and often find their particular way of perceiving and communicating in the world intrusive and exhausting. Here, I am in danger of using the terms 'us' and 'them', or implying that there are the 'mentally ill' and the rest of us are all 'sane'. Of course, as mental health nurses, we are constantly reminded of our own fragmented and disturbing thoughts and feelings. It is just that 'our' way of perceiving and communicating, is deemed as relatively sane by those in charge. Nurses, therefore, need support in their work and this can be achieved to a large extent within the supervisory relationship.

## Supervision and reflective practice

I have attempted to demonstrate in my case studies in Chapter 8, how staff frequently encounter psychical and bodily responses to the patients they work with within mental health practice. These responses are sometimes unsettling and unpleasant. In a supervisory relationship, mental health nurses could discuss how they might feel, as a result of caring for their patients: worn out, violated, anxious, hateful, confused, intruded upon and so on. Alternatively, of course, we also experience joy, humour, and love as a result of working with our patients. It is vital that the supervisor accepts these responses and attempts to encourage the supervisee to acknowledge and make sense of them, in order to understand what is going on for the nurse as well as the patient. In my role as mental health nursing lecturer, I once said to a large group of students that they will at some point in their nursing career feel like killing patients and cutting them up (perhaps I got a little carried away) to which they looked at me in horror. Of course, I am not suggesting that one would *act* upon these feelings (or indeed act upon feelings of love), but, rather, that they should acknowledge them.

Reflective practice is a key term with mental health nursing practice whereby there is emphasis upon learning from experience. Nurses are encouraged to examine what they do and why they do it and for this to inform their future practice. As Sheila Forster suggests: 'By questioning the process of a situation faced in practice, the practitioner is able to take up the opportunity to analyse the situation and the outcome critically and understand what learning and professional development has taken place' (1997: 111). Reflective practice can be held on wards in a group setting among members of a staff team or in one-to-one supervision between two staff members. Reflective practice enables nurses to collectively discuss their experiences of working with patients. This is perhaps a forum whereby the knowledge gained from attention to the body and countertransference issues may be understood and processed. This practice would obviously require staff to be committed to attempting to understand their psychical and physical responses to patients.

## Working with countertransference

Nurses are encouraged to examine their responses when working with patients but, again, specific *bodily* responses are not examined in terms of what they might signify about patients and their experiences. Nurses are taught to pay attention to the body language of their patients in terms of what this might signify in terms of their mental distress. An example of this would be a patient who is withdrawn and curled up in a foetal position and how this might signify that they are depressed. Nurses are not taught to think about and examine their own bodily responses. It would be useful for nurses to realise that their own bodies are brought into their relations with patients. The patient who particularly highlighted this process was Alice, who seemed to bring my body into our interaction. She positioned me in contrast to her as rather insignificant and seemed to perceive me as visible with stature.

Nurses are currently taught the importance of 'self-awareness'. It is considered that through being self-aware nurses could work more effectively with their patients. I consider that attention to countertransference issues – and attention to what psychical processes belong to patients and what belong to the practitioner – can further add to a position of awareness for staff members. I suggest that being aware (of oneself and the patient), in itself, changes the dynamic between the patient and nurse. It is interesting how a very challenging patient can change once an understanding of their effect upon you, or your response to them, is achieved. An example of this is fear. Some patients evoke fear in the staff working with them. However, once the fear is acknowledged and articulated by the staff member, they may begin to understand that perhaps the patient is frightened. Consequently, the dynamic then changes. It is as if the patient then behaves in ways that appear less frightening.

I feel it would also be useful for nurses to acknowledge their feelings of hate and frustration, particularly when working with difficult patients, as theorists including Searles and Winnicott have suggested. As I have stated, these feelings can be acknowledged and understood within the supervisory relationship. Winnicott asserts the necessity of clinical hatred. He goes as far as suggesting that if the analyst cannot hate their patient, the patient cannot tolerate their hate of the analyst. He acknowledges the often emotional burden of working with psychotic people and the often intense emotions, including hatred, they can evoke in the staff working with them. The issue of clinical hatred is rarely acknowledged within mental health nursing practice and warrants further examination.

As I hope my accounts of patients show, there are various physical and psychical responses that emerge when interacting with mental health patients. In my chapter on countertransference, I detailed how theorists have suggested that mental health practitioners experience emotions such as disgust and frustration in their work with people with psychosis, in particular. There is often a sense that these patients are psychically *getting inside* and so forth. As a result of her work with psychotic patients, Little suggested that primitive defence mechanisms are activated in those who work closely with patients with psychosis. We often want to protect ourselves from the feelings evoked in us as a result of working with disturbed people. What I experienced with the men in particular, was a strong psychical and physical sense of their fragmentation. Consequently, I experienced the interviews and the writing up of them, as particularly distressing. In addition, I felt overwhelmed in response to the often disturbing experiences these patients presented to me both verbally and non-verbally. I felt my responses of distress helped me better understand the experiences of these people. However, in addition it is important to note that my responses might also have indicated my wish to detach or protect myself from the feelings evoked in me by these patients. I felt it necessary to process and make sense of these distressing feelings. This highlights the issue of what mental health nurses might do with the insights and knowledge they have acquired about patients through attending to their countertransference responses. Nurses require time to think about the people they care for and to share and make sense of their responses within a safe forum.

## Understanding our patients

In this book I have stressed that, as mental health practitioners, attention to the bodily presentations of patients and our responses to them often help us understand our patients better. I hope I have demonstrated in Chapter 8 that I reached a better understanding of the four patients I observed and interviewed by considering the apparent meanings in their 'symptoms' in the form of bodily expressions, and my reactions to them. How do these insights on the part of the mental health practitioners actually help our patients? I can certainly say that my perceived insights helped me, as I have stated, gain some insight into the needs and experiences of the people I spent time with in relation to their feelings about themselves and their relation to others. My apparent insights also enabled me to go beyond diagnosis, and to think about them as people who are not mere clinical and biological subjects. I am convinced that patients appreciate this effort on the part of the people who care for them.

As I outlined in Chapter 6, Bion suggests that bodily or concrete symptoms, if tolerated and 'held' by the analyst, can be fed back as experiences and thus transformed into more tolerable, thinkable ideas for the patient. In her discussion of countertransference, Little suggests that the patient may, through a therapeutic relationship, be able to introject, or take in, aspects of the analyst's good, integrated ego. Applied to mental health practice, this requires the nurse to stay with the patients in their distress and to bear that distress. In this context it is helpful to be able to differentiate between your feelings and those of the person you are caring for. To overcome this potential difficulty, in the practice of psychoanalysis, the analyst is required to undergo their own analysis in order to become aware of, and take responsibility for, their own feelings and reactions to others. It would, undoubtedly, be useful for nurses to undergo their own analysis in order to make sense of the transference and counter-transference processes in their interactions with patients, and to avoid clinical despair. There would have to be a generally recognised need for this articulated by service commissioners, practitioners and teachers, so that provisions were incorporated structurally within mental health nursing practice.

Working psychodynamically with patients obviously requires an intense and therapeutic approach. I am not suggesting that using a psychodynamic approach in the care of people with mental illness means nurses will *analyse* their patients. It is vital to acknowledge that not everyone wants to return to the past, particularly if there are distressing memories. It would be rather neglectful and abusive to bring painful past experiences to the surface and then just leave the patient with them by failing to offer any further support and contact. I am suggesting that we can at least recognise our patients' expressions as possible indicators of their experience rather than just meaningless signs and symptoms. Through our ability to stay with our patients, through looking at and making sense of our responses, we can gain some insight into how they perceive and relate to the world.

In order for such an approach to nursing practice to be effectively utilised, a psychodynamic understanding of processes between staff and patients has to be an integral part of mental health nurse training and practice. Murray Jackson suggests that developments in the understanding of psychosis from within psychoanalytic theory can be integrated with developments in psychosocial, psychological and pharmacological approaches in nursing. Jackson acknowledges that within a ward environment, it is the mental health nurse who knows the patients best. The skills of the nurse can be used at many levels, from their role as a lead nurse – an essential first point of contact for the patient – through to training as a psychotherapeutic practitioner.

Jackson suggests nurses could be encouraged to stay on mental health units for considerable amounts of time in order to build therapeutic relationships with patients. This would differ considerably from the present situation where there is high turnover of staff. Jackson suggests that nurses, who are given supportive and effective supervisory help and who are well informed about psychoanalytic perspectives of the experience of psychosis, could 'contain' patients by their informed understanding. Jackson is drawing upon Klein's theory of projection that suggests that individuals split off and project out the perceived 'bad' aspects of themselves that they are unable to tolerate. Klein states that this is particularly apparent in the case of psychosis when the ego is severely fragmented. By being calm and 'holding' the experience, or as Bion suggests, by 'containing' them, mental health nurses are responding beneficially to the patient. In this way, the patient may be assured that the nurse has not been destroyed by their projections. Jackson suggests that by maintaining their composure, a nurse may also reduce the anxiety of a patient and this may also result in considerably lower levels of medication being prescribed to patients (2001: 299).

## Actions speak louder than words

As I have stated, following the insights of Klein and Bion, people with psychosis often have difficulty in forming symbols. Therefore, words are often used as actions and things. Words are therefore an ineffective way of communicating for many patients. Therefore, the nurse might try to communicate in a non-verbal way. Perhaps gestures made by the nurse can show the patient that they have been understood. There is a possibility that, within mental health nursing practice, action can be used in the place of words to benefit people who are distressed. Mike Swinburne, a mental health practitioner, outlines that this is the philosophy of a *psycho-social practice* approach. Daily activities – domestic and recreational – are understood in this context as a means of understanding the interactions between staff and patients and as a way of making sense of patients' actions.

Swinburne offers a case study of a patient with schizophrenia who makes a mess in the toilet with his own faeces. In a Kleinian sense, this action may symbolise the split off and projected out aspects of this patient. Swinburne suggests that by actively helping the patient clean up his mess, staff may be able to enable the patient to take some of these projected out fragments back into himself, thus enabling his ego to eventually strengthen (2000: 229). This approach differs from some areas of clinical practice. It is often thought that patients need to break their dependency upon staff. Therefore, there is emphasis upon patients doing activities such as washing themselves or cooking, by themselves in order to be autonomous. This suggests that a patient's mess is not the business of the staff. In contrast, Swinburne's example suggests that the patient's mess is rather an integral part of the patient–practitioner relationship.

## Dance movement therapy

Dance movement therapy (DMT) may be a forum in which psychotic patients may be encouraged to make use of their bodily expression of their experience more effectively. DMT focuses upon the importance of non-verbal bodily expression in communication. Gayle Liebowitz suggests that DMT can effectively be practised within in-patient mental health settings with psychotic patients. She states the importance of focusing upon the early experiences of people with psychosis and proposes that DMT is a valuable treatment in this context. Liebowitz states that in DMT, there is a meeting between the client and therapist, which not only reveals the present situation but also the past. She states that memories of past bodily encounters and experiences are symbolised within the current or present body. DMT therefore aims to bring about connections to these bodily memories and enable the patient to make more sense of them in the present (Liebowitz in Payne 1992: 103).

Liebowitz suggests that many psychotic people have experienced trauma in early life and therefore have not progressed beyond the oral stage. Consequently, they often reveal through bodily means, a lack of a sense of having their feet on the ground, or a lack of an awareness of direction in space (ibid.: 105). Many DMT theorists also specify that in psychosis, there is a lack of unity between the mind and body. Therefore, the aim of working with psychotic patients is to encourage an integrated body image and to strengthen a realistic sense of the body.

This approach can also allow emphasis to be placed upon counter-transference responses in staff. In DMT, this includes attention to bodily as well as psychical responses. Kristina Stanton states that an understanding of the patient's experience can be achieved if the DMT therapist reflects the bodily movements of the patient, 'either with words or with the body of the therapist' (Stanton in ibid.: 124).

## Psychiatry

As I have stated, psychiatrists very usefully pay much attention to the bodily presentations of mental illness in their work with patients, particularly within assessment and diagnostic processes. It seems that this emphasis upon the body is often within a biomedical framework whereby bodily symptoms of mental illness are considered to relate to a specific diagnostic category. In this book, I have suggested that psychiatrists, in their rather powerful position at the top of the mental health hierarchy, often appear to reinforce the biomedical discourses about how mental illness is understood and treated. Perhaps, then, there is little hope of changing the framework within which mental illness is defined.

There are many psychiatrists who consider the meanings apparent in psychiatric symptoms and work sensitively and therapeutically. However, when a person's distress is merely reduced to biological explanations, it does appear that attention to the events of their lives is rather neglected. I am reminded here of a meeting I attended with a psychiatrist and patient. The psychiatrist seemed to pay little attention to this patient's expressions of her lived experiences and instead chose to consider her distress purely within a biomedical framework. The patient had fled to the UK from her country of origin. She had then married a man who was violent towards her and she managed to escape to a women's refuge. She was terrified of her husband coming to get her and she had put on weight, which I considered was an attempt to disguise herself. At times, she heard her husband's voice inside her head. In the meeting I attended, she described to the psychiatrist how a man, as she put it, was 'growing bigger and filling in her head'. The psychiatrist replied by suggesting his disbelief that a man could possibly be inside her head. 'Isn't it rather', he said, 'that it's the chemicals in your brain causing this?'

Psychiatrists tend to see patients when they are initially admitted to hospital in order to assess them and recommend specific interventions. Patients are also regularly seen by psychiatrists for regular meetings to monitor their treatment and progress. It is nurses, perhaps more than any other mental health professional, who spend more time with patients on the day-to-day running of a ward and in other therapeutic settings. I consider that this enables nurses to work with patients in a therapeutic manner.

In this concluding chapter, I have suggested some ways in which awareness of the body in expressing lived experience and the focus upon physical and psychical responses in staff working with mentally ill patients may be incorporated into mental health nursing practice. I started this book with an example of one of my early patients, whom I called Marilyn.

At the time, her bodily presentation was both striking and startling to me. I wondered what her body said about her life. I thought about her statements about disappearing expressed in her apparent fear of her body being sucked up into the sky or washed down the plughole. I thought Marilyn was expressing her needs through her 'symptoms'. It seemed that she wished for her body to be transported – and it didn't feel 'at home' in her new surroundings. Did she want to be in that residential home at all? Were these apparent meaningless 'delusions' related to her wish to escape and be returned to the institution where she formally lived – her home – of which she spoke of frequently?

I have attempted to demonstrate in the case studies in Chapter 8, that the effort to make sense of our patients' bodily presentations is worthwhile. Turan had experienced an orthodox Islamic upbringing and seemed to resist its requirements. Consequently, he felt cursed by his parents who had pressured him to pray. The cursing continued in a concrete manner in the form of hallucinations – in the voices he heard and from people 'lurking' around him. The radioactive metal plate in his leg – a delusion – prevented him from kneeling to pray. His body was a site of psychical conflict.

Tom lost his mother at the age of four in a horrific crash. He felt responsible for this accident but had attempted to forget how guilty and upset he felt. Tom's guilt was reinforced first by his grandmother who seemed to blame him for his mother's death, and then by his godfather who punished him through physical and sexual abuse. He continued to repeat his early experience of being smashed up – so clearly symbolised in his body – so to somehow keep alive and repair the damage he felt he had done.

The women I interviewed, who wondered why, it seemed, I even bothered about them, did not seem to value their own bodies – themselves. Moira experienced her mother's mental illness from an early age as being her fault. This seemed to be confirmed to Moira by the physical abuse she received from her mother. Moira would damage her own body as punishment, and perhaps unintentionally, enable others to hurt her. Alice, too, felt a sense of guilt it seemed from the time she was born. Her mother had experienced complications in pregnancy while carrying her. Alice's guilt was experienced concretely in the form of the cursing voices she heard. She had deadened her feelings of need for others and felt dead inside, as if her body was rotting. The distress of these women appeared to be stuck inside their bodies and was somehow unreachable. While on one hand I felt irritated and deadened by their dismissive perceptions of their own bodies as worthless and their perceived failures as women, it also seemed to me that this very speech was all that was available to them.

Thinking about the meanings within our patients' symptoms often involves focusing upon their past life experiences. However, it has to be acknowledged that people often find the past distressing and do not want to return to it, even if it is clear that they seem to be carrying it with them and it is preventing them from relating to others and functioning in the world. It is also the case that 'talking about it' is not necessarily desirable or effective for all patients. However, in listening to the speech of 'neurotic' patients, in particular the various omissions, evasions and dead ends and so on, practitioners can be led towards the understanding of the significance of past, swallowed down and seemingly forgotten events that the patient has never quite overcome. In this context, the painful, unacceptable idea or thought that has been repressed, comes to the surface and is worked through and potentially resolved through speaking.

However, in the case of psychosis, words frequently do not have the same significance. But we still need to be attentive to the speech of patients and not dismiss it as inappropriate or meaningless. In psychosis, experiences and needs are frequently felt and communicated in a concrete manner as 'things'. These various expressions, so often presented through the body – and I have offered some examples in my case studies in Chapter 8 – are worth acknowledging and feeling. In this way, we may begin to bring the body more fully into mental health practice, and thereby look beyond diagnosis towards a richer understanding of the feelings and needs of the people who are in our care.

# Notes

## 1 Introduction

1 See, for example, Orbach, S. *Fat is a Feminist Issue* (Arrow Books 1988); Lawrence, M. *Fed Up and Hungry* (The Women's Press 1987); and Roth, G. *Breaking Free from Compulsive Eating* (Grafton Books 1986) for discussions relating to eating disorders. Marilee Strong in *A Bright Red Scream: Self Mutilation and the Language of Pain* (Penguin 1998) provides a comprehensive discussion of self-harm and includes real-life portraits of people who self-harm.
2 See, for example, Katherine Phillips *The Broken Mirror: Understanding and Treating Body Dysmorphic Disorder* (Oxford University Press 1998).
3 After much consideration, I have decided to use the term 'bodily presentation' rather than, say, 'bodily expression' – in the hope that it does not sound too clinical.
4 With the exception of more recent theorists including Teresa Brennan and Elizabeth Grosz, both discussed in this book.

## 2 Lived experience

1 For selected writings by Descartes, see Cottingham (1996).

## 3 Bodily inscription

1 The first appearance of this paper was in *Hommage a Jean Hyppolite* (Paris: Presses Universitaires de France, 1971, pp. 145–72). Rabinow in *The Foucault Reader* (1984), asserts that this paper is essential in the understanding of Foucault's objectives and the later development of his work.
2 The American version of the *ICD-10* is the *DSM* (*Diagnostic and Statistical Manual of Mental Disorders*).
3 This textbook ceased to be in print from January 2001. However, it has continued to be used by training mental health nurses as a reference book.

## 4 Women speaking

1 See, for example, Price and Shildrick (1999) and Schiebinger (2000) for comprehensive writings on the body and feminism.
2 See, for example, the chapter on women, the body and depression by Stoppard in Ussher (1997). Stoppard examines how depression in women has been understood and treated within a biomedical framework. She stresses that it is also

important to understand the ways in which the symptoms of depression have been constructed within culture as essentially relating to women.

3 In my original PhD study, I interviewed another two women patients who also spoke of factors relating to care of others, isolation and guilt at not being a 'good enough' mother and wife. It seemed that these issues largely contributed to their distress (and this has often seemed apparent in the many women patients I have worked with during the past nineteen years).

4 For a discussion of biomedical explanations of women's mental illness, see, for example, Russell (1995).

5 Ulrich, H. (1987) 'A Study of Change and Depression among Havik Brahmin Women in a South Indian Village', *Culture, Medicine and Psychiatry*, vol. 11, pp. 261–87

6 I use the terms 'mad' or 'madness' in this section, as these are the terms Chesler and Showalter use.

## 6 Psychosis

1 Kristeva outlines her use of the term 'chora' to describe the circulation of drives in her essay, 'Revolution in Poetic Language', in Moi (1986), p. 93.

2 In her book *Mothering Psychoanalysis* (1992), Janet Sayers describes how Melanie Klein's daughter Melitta had referred to her mother as controlling and intrusive.

3 Winnicott makes much more of the importance of the maternal environment. See, for example, 'The Development of the Capacity for Concern', in *The Maturational Processes and the Facilitating Environment* (New York: International Universities Press, 1965, pp. 73–82).

## 7 The practitioner's body

1 Freud states he has borrowed the term 'imago' from Jung, e.g. 'father-imago'.

## 8 The patient's body

1 See, for example, 'Gay and Lesbian Identities and Mental Health' in Kelleher and Leavey (2004).

# Bibliography

Barrett, M. (1980) *Women's Oppression Today*, London: Verso.

Bartky, S. (1990) *Femininity and Domination: Studies in the Phenomenology of Oppression*, New York: Routledge.

Bion, W.R. (1992) *Cogitations*, London: Karnac Books.

Bion, W.R. (1993) *Second Thoughts*, London: Karnac Books.

Bowie, M. (1991) *Lacan*, London: Fontana Press.

Breggin, P. (1993) *Toxic Psychiatry: Drugs and Electroconvulsive Therapy: The Truth and the Better Alternatives*, London: Fontana.

Brennan, T. (1992) *The Interpretation of the Flesh: Freud and Femininity*, London: Routledge.

Brooking, J.I., Ritter, S.A. and Thomas, B.L. (eds) (1992) *A Textbook of Psychiatric and Mental Health Nursing*, London: Churchill Livingstone.

Brown, G.W. and Harris, T. (1978) *Social Origins of Depression: A Study of Psychiatric Disorder in Women*, London: Tavistock.

Busfield, J. (1996) *Men, Women and Madness*, London: Macmillan.

Cameron, D. (1985) *Feminism and Linguistic Theory*, New York: St Martin's Press.

Campbell, D. and Stanley, J. (1963) *Experimental and Quasi-experimental Designs for Research*, Chicago, IL: Rand McNally.

Chesler, P. (1997) *Women and Madness*, New York: Four Walls, Eight Windows.

Chodorow, N. (1978) *The Reproduction of Mothering*, London: University of California Press.

Cormack, D.F.S. (ed.) (2000) *The Research Process in Nursing*, Oxford: Blackwell.

Cottingham, J. (ed.) (1996) *Descartes: Meditations on First Philosophy: With Selections from the Objections and Replies*, London: Cambridge University Press.

Darwin, C. (1883) *The Descent of Man and Selection in Relation to Sex*, New York: Appleton.

David-Menard, M. (1989) *Hysteria from Freud to Lacan: The Body and Language in Psychoanalysis*, Ithaca, NY: Cornell University Press.

Day, T. (1993) *More Like Home: The Story of Long Grove Hospital and How It Was Closed to Improve Mental Health Services*, Kingston and Esher Health Authority.

Department of Health (2003) *Mainstreaming Gender and Women's Mental Health*, London: DH.

Diamond, I. and Quinby, L. (eds) (1988) *Femininity and Foucault: Reflections on Resistance*, Boston, MA: Northeastern University Press.

Doane, J. and Hodges, D. (1992) *From Klein to Kristeva: Psychoanalytic Feminism and the Search for the 'Good Enough Mother'*, Ann Arbor, MI: The University of Michigan Press.

Doyal, L. (1995) *What Makes Women Sick?*, London: Macmillan.

Dworkin, A. (1979) *Pornography: Men Possessing Women*, London: The Women's Press.

Ellwood, J. (ed.) (1995) *Psychosis: Understanding and Treatment*, London: Jessica Kingsley Publishers.

Evans, D. (1996) *An Introductory Dictionary of Lacanian Psychoanalysis*, London: Routledge.

Featherstone, M., Hepworth, M. and Turner, B.S. (eds) (1991) *The Body: Social Process and Cultural Theory*, London: Sage.

Firestone, S. (1970) *The Dialectic of Sex*, New York: Bantam Books.

Foreman, A. (1977) *Femininity as Alienation: Women and the Family in Marxism and Psychoanalysis*, London: Pluto Press.

Forster, S. (1997) *The A-Z of Community Mental Health Practice*, Cheltenham: Nelson Thornes (Publishers) Ltd.

Foucault, M. (1954, revised in 1962) *Mental Illness and Psychology*, London: University of California Press.

Foucault, M. (1965) *Madness and Civilisation: A History of Insanity in the Age of Reason*, London: Routledge.

Foucault, M. (1977) *Discipline and Punish: The Birth of the Prison*, London: Penguin.

Foucault, M. (1990) *The History of Sexuality: Volume 1, An Introduction*, London: Penguin.

Freud, S. (1894) 'The Neuro-Psychoses of Defence', in *The Standard Edition of the Complete Psychological Works of Sigmund Freud* (SE), London: The Hogarth Press, vol. 3.

Freud, S. (1895a) *Project for a Scientific Psychology*, SE 1.

Freud, S. (1895b) *The Psychotherapy of Hysteria*, SE 2.

Freud, S. (1896) *The Aetiology of Hysteria*, SE 3.

Freud, S. (1900) *The Interpretation of Dreams*, SE 4.

Freud, S. (1905a) *Fragment of an Analysis of a Case of Hysteria*, SE 7.

Freud, S. (1905b) *Three Essays on the Theory of Sexuality*, SE 7.

Freud, S. (1908) *On the Sexual Theories of Children*, SE 9.

Freud, S. (1910) *The Future Prospects of Psycho-Analytic Therapy*, SE 11.

Freud, S. (1911a) *Psycho-Analytic Notes on an Autobiographical Account of a Case of Paranoia*, SE 12.

Freud, S. (1911b) 'On the Mechanism of Paranoia', SE 12.

Freud, S. (1912) *The Dynamics of Transference*, SE 12.

Freud, S. (1913) 'The Disposition to Obsessional Neurosis', SE 12.

Freud, S. (1914a) *On Narcissism: An Introduction*, SE 14.

Freud, S. (1914b) *Remembering, Repeating and Working-Through*, SE 12.

Freud, S. (1914c) *Observations on Transference-Love*, SE 12.

Freud, S. (1917a) 'Psycho-Analysis and Psychiatry', SE 16.

Freud, S. (1917b) 'The Sense of Symptoms', SE 16.

Freud, S. (1917c) 'The Paths to the Formation of Symptoms', SE 16.

Freud, S. (1923) *The Ego and the Id*, SE 19.

Freud, S. (1924a) 'Neurosis and Psychosis', SE 19.

Freud, S. (1924b) *The Loss of Reality in Neurosis and Psychosis*, SE 19.

Freud, S. (1924c) *The Dissolution of the Oedipus Complex*, SE 19.

Freud, S. (1925) *Some Psychical Consequences of the Anatomical Distinction Between the Sexes*, SE 19.

Freud, S. (1933) 'Femininity', SE 22.

Freud, S. (1984) *On Metapsychology*, London: Penguin.

Freud, S. (1986) *The Essentials of Psychoanalysis,* London: Penguin.

Freud, S. and Breuer, J. (1895) *Studies on Hysteria*, SE 2.

Gay, P. (1988) *Freud: A Life for Our Time*, London: Papermac.

Gelder, M., Gath, D. and Cowan, P. (2001) *Shorter Oxford Dictionary of Psychiatry*, New York: Oxford University Press.

Glaser, B.G. and Strauss, A.C. (1967) *The Discovery of Grounded Theory: Strategies for Qualitative Research*, New York: Aldine.

Granville, M.J. (1877) *Care and Cure of the Insane,* London: Hardwick and Bogue.

Grosz, E. (1990) *Jacques Lacan: A Feminist Introduction*, London: Routledge.

Grosz, E. (1994) *Volatile Bodies: Toward a Corporeal Feminism*, Bloomington, IN: Indiana University Press.

Gunew, S. (ed.) (1991) *A Reader in Feminist Knowledge*, London: Routledge.

Hamblet, C. (2000) 'Obstacles to Defining the Role of the Mental Health Nurse', *Nursing Standard*, 6 September, vol. 14, no. 5.

Hartmann, H. (1981) *The Unhappy Marriage of Marxism and Feminism*, London: Pluto Press.

Hinshelwood, R.D. (1991) *A Dictionary of Kleinian Thought*, London: Free Association.

Holmstrom, N. (1984) 'A Marxist Theory of Women's Nature', *Ethics* 94, no. 1: 464.

Hudson, D. (1987) 'You Can't Commit Violence Against an Object: Women, Psychiatry and Psychosurgery', in Jalna Hanmer and Mary Maynard (eds), *Women, Violence and Social Control*, London: Macmillan Press.

Hunter, D. (1983) 'Hysteria, Psychoanalysis, and Feminism: The Case of Anna "O"', *Feminist Studies* 9, no. 3.

Husserl, E. (2001) *Logical Investigations, Volume 1*, London: Routledge.

Irigaray, L. (1977) 'Women's Exile', *Ideology and Consciousness*, 1: 74.

Irigaray, L. (1985a) *Speculum of the Other Woman*, New York: Cornell University Press.

Irigaray, L. (1985b) *This Sex Which is Not One*, New York: Cornell University Press.

Jackson, M. (2001) *Weathering the Storms: Psychotherapy for Psychosis*, London: Karnac.

Jones, C. and Porter, R. (eds) (1994) *Reassessing Foucault: Power, Medicine and the Body*, London: Routledge.

Kafka, F. (1986) *Metamorphosis and Other Stories*, London: Penguin.

Kelleher, D. and Leavey, G. (2004) *Identity and Health*, London: Routledge.

Klein, M. (1997) *The Psychoanalysis of Children*, London: Vintage.

Klein, M., Heimann, P., Issacs, S. and Riviere, J. (1955) *Developments in Psychoanalysis*, London: Hogarth.

Knapp, T. (1998) *Quantitative Nursing Research*, London: Sage.

Kristeva, J. (1987) *Tales of Love*, New York: Columbia University Press.

Kristeva, J. (1995) *New Maladies of the Soul*, New York: Columbia University Press.

Lacan, J. (1977) *Ecrits: A Selection*, London: Tavistock.

Laing, R.D. (1969) *The Divided Self*, London: Penguin Books.

Laplanche, J. and Pontalis, J.B. (1988) *The Language of Psychoanalysis*, London: Karnac.

Little, M. (1951) 'Counter-transference and the Patient's Response to It', *International Journal of Psychoanalysis*, 32.

McDougall, J. (1989) *Theatres of the Body: A Psychoanalytic Approach to Psychosomatic Illness*, London: Free Association.

McNay, L. (1992) *Foucault and Feminism*, London: Polity Press.

Malcolm, J. (1992) *The Purloined Clinic: Selected Writings*, New York: Papermac.

Marx, K. and Engels, F. (1967) *The Communist Manifesto*, London: Penguin.

Masson J.M. (1985) *The Complete Letters of Sigmund Freud to Wilhelm Fliess 1887–1904*, Cambridge, MA: Harvard University Press.

Miles, A. (1988) *Women and Mental Illness*, Brighton: Wheatsheaf.

Millett, K. (1970) *Sexual Politics*, London: Virago.

Minsky, R. (1996) *Psychoanalysis and Gender*, London: Routledge.

Mitchell, J. (1971) *Women's Estate*, New York: Pantheon Books.

Mitchell, J. (1986) *The Selected Melanie Klein*, London: Penguin.

Mitchell, J. and Rose, J. (1982) (eds) *Feminine Sexuality: Jacques Lacan and the Ecole Freudienne*, New York: Norton.

Moi, T. (1986) *The Kristeva Reader*, Oxford: Blackwell.

Nieswiadomy, R.M. (1998) *Foundations of Nursing Research*, Stamford, CT: Appleton & Lange.

Nietzsche, F. (1996) *On the Genealogy of Morals*, Oxford: Oxford University Press.

Oakley, A. (1974) *Housewife: High Value, Low Cost*, London: Penguin.

Oppenheim, A.N. (1992) 'Standardised Interviews', *Questionnaire Design, Interviewing and Attitude Measurement*, London: Pinter.

Orbach, S. (1999) *The Impossibility of Sex*, London: Allen Lane The Penguin Press.

Padel, R. (1995) *Whom Gods Destroy: Elements of Greek and Tragic Madness*, Princeton, NJ: Princeton University Press.

Payne, H. (1992) *Dance Movement Therapy: Theory and Practice*, London: Routledge.

Plato (1977) *Timaeus and Cirtias*, London: Penguin.

Porter, R. (2002) *Madness: A Brief History*, New York: Oxford University Press.

Price, J. and Shildrick, M. (1999) *Feminist Theory and the Body*, Edinburgh: Edinburgh University Press.

Rabinow, P. (ed.) (1984) *The Foucault Reader*, London: Penguin.

Rich, A. (1976) *Of Woman Born*, London: Virago.

Rosenfeld, H. (1952a) 'Notes on the Psycho-Analysis of the Super-Ego Conflict in an Acute Catatonic Patient', *International Journal of Psychoanalysis*: 33.

Rosenfeld, H. (1952b) 'Transference-Phenomena and Transference-Analysis in an Acute Catatonic Patient', *International Journal of Psychoanalysis*: 33.

Rowbotham, S. (1973) *Woman's Consciousness, Man's World*, London: Pelican Books.

Russell, D. (1995) *Women, Madness and Medicine*, London: Polity.

Sayers, J. (1992) *Mothering Psychoanalysis*, London: Penguin.

Sayers, J. (2000) *Kleinians: Psychoanalysis Inside Out*, London: Polity.

Schilder, P. (1976) *On Psychoses*, New York: International Universities Press.

Schiebinger, L. (2000) *Feminism and the Body*, New York: Oxford University Press.

Schilder, P. (1978) *The Image and Appearance of the Human Body*, New York: International University Press.

Searles, H.F. (1964) *Collected Papers on Schizophrenia and Related Papers*, New York: International University Press.

Sechehaye, Marguerite (ed.) (1951) *Autobiography of a Schizophrenic Girl* (trans. from 1950 French edn), New York: New American Library.

Segal, H. (1981) *The Work of Hanna Segal*, New York: Jason Aronson.

Segal, J. (1992) *Melanie Klein*, London: Sage.

Shilling, C. (1993) *The Body and Social Theory*, London: Sage.

Shorter, E. (1997) *A History of Psychiatry: From the Era of the Asylum to the Age of Prozac*, New York: John Wiley & Sons.

Showalter, E. (1985) *The Female Malady: Women, Madness and English Culture, 1830–1980*, London: Virago.

Showalter, E. (1998) *Hystories: Hysterical Epidemics and Modern Culture*, New York: Picador.

Slavney, P.R. (1990) *Perspectives on Hysteria*, Baltimore, MD: Johns Hopkins University Press.

Stone, M.H. (1997) *Healing the Mind: A History of Psychiatry from Antiquity to the Present*, London: Pimlico.

Swinburne, M. (2000) 'Home Is Where the Hate Is', *Psychoanalytic Psychotherapy*, vol. 14, no. 3.

Symington, J. and Symington, N. (1996) *The Clinical Thinking of Wilfred Bion*, London: Routledge.

Thompson, T. and Mathias, P. (2000) *Lyttle's Mental Health and Disorder*, London: Bailliere Tindall.

Tong, R. (1989) *Feminist Thought: A Comprehensive Introduction*, London: Routledge.

Turner, B.S. (1984) *The Body and Society: Explorations in Social Theory*, Oxford: Basil Blackwell.

Turner, B.S. (1992) *Regulating Bodies: Essays in Medical Sociology*, London: Routledge.

Ussher, J.M. (ed.) (1997) *Body Talk: The Material and Discursive Regulation of Sexuality, Madness and Reproduction*, London: Routledge.

Veith, I. (1965) *Hysteria: The History of a Disease*, Chicago, IL: The University of Chicago Press.

Watkins, P. (2001) *Mental Health Nursing: The Art of Compassionate Care*, Edinburgh: Butterworth Heinemann.

Weiss, G. (1999) *Body Images: Embodiment as Intercorporeality*, London: Routledge.

Welton, D. (ed.) (1999) *The Body*, Oxford: Blackwell.

Whitford, M. (ed.) (1991) *The Irigaray Reader*, Oxford: Blackwell.

Williams, J., Watson, G., Smith, G., Copperman, J. and Wood, D. (1993) *Purchasing Effective Mental Health Services for Women: A Framework for Action*, London: Mind Publishers.

Winnicott, D. (1965) *The Maturational Processes and the Facilitating Environment*, New York: International University Press.

Winnicott, D.W. (1984) *Through Paediatrics to Psychoanalysis: Collected Papers*, London: Karnac.

WHO (1993) *The ICD-10 Classification of Mental and Behavioural Disorders*, Geneva: World Health Organisation.

Wright, E. (1984) *Psychoanalytic Criticism: Theory in Practice*, New York: Methuen.

# Index